University of Missouri Press   Columbia and London

BROKEN
Butterfly

BROKEN *Butterfly*

My Daughter's
Struggle with Brain Injury

Karin Finell

Copyright © 2012 by
The Curators of the University of Missouri
University of Missouri Press, Columbia, Missouri 65201
Printed and bound in the United States of America
All rights reserved
5 4 3 2 1   16 15 14 13 12

Cataloging-in-Publication data available from the Library of Congress.
ISBN 978-0-8262-1993-0

∞™ This paper meets the requirements of the
American National Standard for Permanence of Paper
for Printed Library Materials, Z39.48, 1984.

Design and composition: Jennifer Cropp
Printing and binding: Thomson-Shore, Inc.
Typefaces: Minion, Rapier, MS Reference Sans Serif, and Myriad Pro

I am the keeper of fragile things and I
have kept of you what is indissolvable.

—*Anaïs Nin*

Vision is the art of seeing the invisible.

—*Jonathan Swift*

Contents

BUTTERFLY

Actually I had a butterfly come through
my window one time and land
on my shoulder.
That is not a lie.
A yellow butterfly
Right on me.
Shhh! I said.
It made me so happy.
I love butterflies. And birds.
Mostly butterflies.
I love their softness and grace.
In the garden I call, Butterfly, Butterfly.
I like to see them flying
through the sky when it's a little breezy,
a gentle breeze, not hard, when the trees sway
softly.

Butterflies are free
But they don't live very long.
There is one.
I am blown away.

—Stephanie Finell, August 9, 1994

Acknowledgments

I met Anaïs Nin a few months before Stephanie was hospitalized. When she heard of Stephanie's illness, she advised me to make a habit of writing the day's events down every night, before memory threw a veil over the activities. She said to record the conversations between the doctors and myself; to note every detail of the surroundings, and most important, the flux of my emotions. I followed her advice, and the first half of this memoir is based on those journal pages. In this book I not only want to give thanks to the writers and editors who helped shape these pages, but since it contains the essence of Stephanie's life, I'd like to thank the many individuals who played an important part in her life and in this story.

This book is the product of the University of Missouri Press, and I cannot thank its staff enough. Foremost is its editor-in-chief, Clair Willcox. Thank you so much, Clair.

I am enormously grateful to my editor, Sara Davis. She deserves a medal for working with my sometimes convoluted Germanic sentence structure. Along with the edits, Sara sifted through many photos to use or discard. All this under the pressure of a tight schedule. Sara, you are a "Wonder Woman!" Beverly Jarrett, former director, years ago encouraged my completion of this book. I thank her for her interest which spurred me on. Beth Chandler deserves kudos for her patience with me. She always answered my questions when, at times, I made a pest of myself. Thank you, Beth. Lyn Smith and Jennifer Gravley have been extremely helpful, and I thank them.

There were numerous doctors who treated Stephanie. My gratitude goes to all of them. I thank Dr. Robert Podosin, pediatric neurologist, for the care he gave my daughter through the years from 1970 to 1994. Stephanie's doctors in Santa Barbara were equally caring, with Dr. Ralph Quijano, her gynecologist, functioning in many roles and as advisor beyond his specialty. Dr. David Agnew took over Stephanie's neurological care in Santa Barbara and renewed our hopes. Dr. Richard Danson was our family internist. All were kind and caring.

The Marianne Frostig Center of Educational Therapy became our lifeline in the summer of 1971. Dr. Frostig, the founder of the Frostig Center, took Stephanie under her tutelage when no other school could be found. Stephanie relearned language, and her life became one of hope. I cannot thank Marianne Frostig enough for the interest she showed and the love she gave to my daughter.

Louise Fields and coteacher Judy Nason, who were Stephanie's teachers in remedial classes at Santa Barbara City College, advised Stephanie to visit Jodi House, which provided counsel and information for those with brain injuries. Here Stephanie met others who had suffered similar damage, all sharing the problems of their often "invisible" illness. My thanks go to this wonderful organization.

Through Jodi House, Stephanie met Renée van Horne and Libby Whaley, who helped Stephanie in various ways. With Libby she went skiing at Big Bear Mountain with other disabled persons. Thank you, Renée and Libby; through you Stephanie experienced a feeling of freedom in the snow and whizzing down a mountain. Also through Jodi House, Stephanie began therapeutic riding at Elaine Kay's Toro Canyon facility. Through Elaine, Stephanie came to participate in the Special Olympics. Thank you, Elaine, for having expanded Stephanie's life to include the world of horses and animals in a deeper sense.

Pat Morales, then principal of Peabody Charter School, accepted the certificate Stephanie had earned, and Stephanie began as a volunteer teacher's aide in K-Grade. Stephanie loved feeling needed by children. Thank you, Pat Morales.

I owe a debt of gratitude to the Santa Barbara Writers Conference, and especially its founder, Barnaby Conrad. The Africa chapters in this book are his favorites. Also at the conference, a former Los Angeles Times book critic, Charles Champlin, surprised me when he was visibly moved by my reading. He encouraged me to finish the book. Thank you, Charles. At the conference, I met Perie Longo, who teaches poetry and is also a licensed psychologist. I arranged for her to meet Stephanie who had not tolerated "standard" therapy but loved this poetry-based therapy and blossomed. Thank you, Perie, for having given Stephanie the tools to take away the pain of loss she felt over her father, and to fill her last months with the beauty of poetry. Marianne Frostig was the first teacher of importance in Stephanie's life, and Perie proved to be the last.

Cork Millner and Grace Rachow gave the pages their first edits. Thank you both. The Thursday Writers have steered me away from emotional outbursts and purple prose. Thank you all: Susan Chiavelli, Susan Gulbransen, Frances Davis, Linda Stewart-Oaten, Janis Jennings, Sheila Tenold, Carrie Brown, and Toni Lorien.

My special thanks go to Dr. David Agnew and Dr. Spencer Nadler who read the text for medical accuracies.

And last, but most important, I thank my husband, Martin, for his daily support. He helped me in untold ways, reading the pages, correcting word choices, or when I felt tense, massaging my neck or bringing me a mug of hot chocolate.

BROKEN *Butterfly*

Chapter One

The Thunderbolt

Life is a lesson to be learned.
—Stephanie Finell

It all began with the bite of a mosquito. Yes, with a bite of this pesky but seemingly so innocuous little insect that sucked her blood. Not just one, but hundreds punctured her arms and legs with red marks that later swelled to small welts. Who would ever have thought that our family's life would become derailed, that its tightly woven fabric would eventually fray and break—all from the bite of a mosquito?

Friday, December 11, 1970

I checked my watch. Eight-fifteen. The school bus was late when it pulled up at the curb. Stephanie's slightly older brother, Steven skipped down the red brick steps and, running toward the bus, saw me at the bathroom window. He waved. I blew him a kiss and waved back. Marvin had already left for the office, scheduled to be in court in downtown Los Angeles by nine. Stephanie, a month past her seventh birthday and still recovering from the *turista* stomach flu she contracted on our recent visit to Mexico, sat in our bed, watching *I Love Lucy*.

I thought of how Stephanie's eyes had sparkled the previous afternoon in anticipation of our plans for this day, a "mother and daughter" day of shopping, lunch in the tearoom at Bullocks Wilshire, and if Steffi felt up to it, perhaps a movie in the afternoon. It was Friday, and I wanted her to stay out of school for one more day. She still felt weak from the Mexican intestinal disorder, but I hoped she would feel better than she had last night. Even then she had

1

insisted she dress and participate in the annual Brownie holiday show at El Rodeo, the school she and Steven attended. Last night, on stage, Stephanie's color suddenly drained to deadly pale. Even the waves in her brown-gold hair went limp. She and her group were on stage singing, "My Heart Belongs to Daddy—" but Stephanie did not finish the song. Stephanie, who loved to sing, dance, act and clown, left the stage and fell into my arms, whispering, "Take me home, Mommy, please—"

The rumbling of a truck broke my thoughts. Through the window I saw it come to a halt in front of our house. Ah, the Christmas tree the four of us had selected before the Brownie performance. Steven played a big part in finding the right tree and looked forward to helping decorate it this evening. Celia, our housekeeper, opened the front door to receive the tree and the sound of bells rang through the house. The Austrian chimes on the front door played "Edelweiss, Edelweiss."

The melody made me smile, and the nostalgic warmth still lingered when I crossed the room to the walk-in closet behind our bed. I heard someone on the television chant, "Meeses Ricardo?"

My hand on the half-opened closet door, I asked, "Steffi, do you have your list for Santa Claus ready?"

Turning, I froze.

Stephanie sat flailing.

Her right side twitched, her body shook, her eyes rolled up into her skull.

I took hold of her, "Stephanie, Stephanie!"

I wrapped my arms around her, held her tight.

Her right leg kicked me as it shot upward. Sheet and blanket pulled off, her body jerked, went stiff, limp, stiff, limp.

She stretched, balanced on head and feet, her torso an arc. Her soft brown eyes were replaced by two white orbs.

"Estefani!"

Celia heard my screech, tossed the Christmas tree onto the terrace, and was by our side. "Que pasó? Que pasó mi niña?"

When she saw what was happening, she sank to her knees next to me. Her hand clasped her mouth. Her eyes brimmed with tears. She made the sign of the cross.

To me, the room and Stephanie appeared as if through mosquito netting. While Celia held my child, I grabbed the phone and dialed: the doctor, my husband's office, my mother. Voices blurred. My eyes tried to regain focus, while Stephanie lay twitching, wrenching, quivering, rigid, limp, rigid, limp, in a relentless spin of random movement.

"It's an emergency, yes," I heard my voice, now a rasp, shriek into the phone. "I have to talk to Dr. Rosin, *now!*" I chewed on my knuckles.

Then a cool, calming voice came over the line. "This is Dr. Rosin."

Why couldn't he be *here, now,* I thought, instead of wasting time on the phone. I tried to concentrate, to be logical, and to speak coherently.

"Wash her down with half alcohol and warm water?" I repeated the doctor's words. Why? I told him she didn't seem to have a temperature. With my voice barely audible I said, "I'm afraid she's dying. I'm not a hysterical mother. You know me." I implored him to come.

His response was *No.* His reception room was filled with patients. He would ask his partner, Dr. Brown, to stop at our house on his way back from the hospital. It made no sense to me, Dr. Brown was at the Cedars of Lebanon Hospital, on Fountain Avenue in Hollywood, a drive of at least fifty minutes. Dr. Rosin's office on Linden and Wilshire was no more than a seven-minute drive from our house.

I returned to Stephanie's side, stroked her hair, matted and wet, my tears mingling with her sweat. Celia brought a bowl filled with equal parts of water and alcohol. We washed Stephanie, though she didn't feel hot. The task filled the vacuum of time. My mother appeared in the room. She had entered the house through the back door. She saw the convulsing body of her grandchild and came to me softly. She clasped me in her arms. My body twitched, small reflexive movements imitating Stephanie's.

The doorbell rang. I jumped. The doctor? Celia ran down to open the door. And again the chimes played "Edelweiss." The notes sounded off-key, the music jarred. I covered my ears to block out the sound.

Where is Marvin? Didn't he get my message? Has he already left for court? I became more frantic. The shadows around me grew darker.

A smiling face appeared in the doorway, Dr. Harold Brown. I had no sense of time, but reasoned an hour must have passed. He looked at Stephanie. The smile dropped from his cheeks. His kind brown eyes grew large behind his tortoiseshell glasses. His legs seemed to be made of rubber, spanning the space as if with one giant step when he reached for her pulse. His left hand fumbled within his medical bag as he fished out a tongue depressor and pushed it into Stephanie's mouth. Then he brought out a syringe and ampoules. "We have to calm her," he said as if to himself. He extracted the liquid, filled the syringe, and checked the clear serum against the light of the window.

I squirmed at the slowness of it all as he checked the syringe *again.* My entire body felt prickly, itching. *Inject her! Calm her! Please!*

He went on with his procedure, pulled the tourniquet tightly around Stephanie's arm, then he injected the needle into her vein. A minute passed. He looked at me. The Phenobarbital hadn't stopped the convulsions.

I listened to the sound I thought to be my husband's car turning into our driveway. Then I heard footsteps leaping up the stairs taking two risers at a time. "Marv. Thank God you're home." I ran to him when he appeared in the doorway. Looking at his face I could read his thoughts: disbelief, shock, then horror when the scene registered. Stephanie's arms flailing like windmills. Her long wavy hair stuck to her head in a tangled, sweaty mass. And her eyes, her lovely dark eyes, were showing only white.

I wondered, *How can her eyes turn up into the skull like this? This only happens in horror movies, not here, not in our bed, not with our child.*

Dr. Brown sat by Stephanie's side, the syringe poised to inject her with a second dose. Her mouth foamed. Her nostrils bubbled greenish mucous.

"We have to calm her. The first dose wasn't strong enough," Dr. Brown turned to address Marvin.

"What . . .What is it. . .She?"

"I don't know, yet. But she's in danger of cardiac arrest if the seizures are too violent."

I hid my head in Marvin's shoulders. He clasped me tight, so tight I could hardly breathe.

"Sorry it took so long. They gave me your message when I arrived at court," he whispered.

I was not aware of how long it had been. Time seemed to run backward and forward simultaneously.

The boundaries between Stephanie's body and mine had evaporated. I was not sure where hers left off and my own began. I felt the flailing, the convulsions as though they were mine.

Marvin and I stood in silence. We watched the doctor's every move—observed his hand, the syringe, the needle lifting and moving toward Stephanie's arm, the needle entering her arm, the liquid slowly emptying into her bloodstream.

This second dose finally calmed her limbs. Small spasms shuddered through her body. Then she grew rigid. Stiff. Very stiff. My hand flew to my mouth. *What?*

Chapter Two

In Limbo

Stephanie was alive.

Dr. Brown and we took separate cars and were to meet at the hospital. To call an ambulance would have taken too long.

Marvin drove. I sat in the passenger's seat holding Stephanie on my lap. Her small child's body seemed, in some bizarre way, like a leaden weight on this surreal ride to the hospital—on the mad rush through amber lights turning red, the eternity we waited for a pedestrian to take his slow ponderous right of way, while I, with every nerve in my body pushed the car to go onward, fast, faster.

The car screeched east on Sunset Boulevard. I noticed the garish billboards flashing topless and bottomless dancers on Sunset Strip. Strange. I wanted not to look, yet I stared at images of naked breasts and grossly exaggerated bare bottoms, growing larger and larger. They mocked my sick child and me. The images whizzed by and disappeared behind us when we turned onto Fountain Avenue.

We reached the hospital in what seemed like hours. Or was it minutes? Time expanded. Time contracted.

Dr. Brown stood waiting at the entrance. Marvin carried Stephanie into the emergency room. A young intern directed us into a small office and fired questions at us.

"Did she have access to drugs? Perhaps in school? LSD? Family history: any brain tumors? Epilepsy? Brain hemorrhage?"

The questions spun in my head. My stomach churned. I wanted to run to the emergency room to be with Stephanie. My repetitive answers sounded as if I were speaking through wads of cotton. "No, no, no—"

The room was small. Stephanie lay in a crib-like bed on a blanket resembling sheep's fleece. An IV attached to her arm dripped a clear liquid into her veins, slowly: drip, drip, drip. A black box behind the bed monitored her heart. Green spikes, a line, another spike showed the rhythm of her seven-year-old heart, connecting her to life. She was alive.

A large window separated Stephanie's room from the nurse's station. I saw the comforting full-moon face of a nurse peering through the glass, watching.

The day's light grew dim. The low sun painted apricot patterns on the white of the woolly fleece and sparked a play of gold in Stephanie's hair, no longer wet from perspiration.

I became aware of the passage of time. *How long have I been here? Where's Marvin?*

There had been endless rounds of tests. I followed the gurney from one examining room to another, down long gray-green corridors. I walked as if I were pushing my way through ever-thickening liquid, viscous like mud. Later I sat on Naugahyde chairs, waiting, waiting.

Marvin paced, sucking on his big Dunhill cigar. At one point he stuck the lighted end into his mouth, grimaced, and spat out the ashes.

I glanced at my watch when he and Dr. Brown asked me to step outside, where we were joined by Dr. Rosin.

I felt like Christopher Isherwood who had compared himself to a camera when he described what he witnessed in Berlin. I was now the camera that took snapshots of the two doctors. They stood as if framed by my Nikon in my viewfinder, and my mind recorded their images. Dr. Rosin appeared as a figure in steel-blue—from his eyes, his metal framed glasses, to the color of his gabardine suit. He cracked his knuckles, increasing my nervousness. The expression on his face reflected a studied solemnity. Dr. Brown's name was echoed in his appearance—in his hair—from his tweed jacket to a well-chewed briar pipe, unlit, which he relentlessly moved from one corner of his mouth to the other. Marvin's thinning hair stood up as if he had seen a ghost. His Acapulco tan had faded within days into gray-beige. His suit looked crumpled, slept in, as if his emotional state manifested itself in his clothes, and his off-center tie hung around his neck like a noose.

"Stephanie is heavily sedated," said Dr. Brown. "We were finally able to calm her."

"You must realize," Dr. Rosin added, "Stephanie is gravely ill. She has quieted down only because of massive doses of Phenobarbital." He turned to Marvin and continued, "Dr. Andler is arranging for an EEG tomorrow." He noticed our puzzled expressions and explained. "Your partner arranged for Dr. Andler to be consulted."

"*The* Dr. Andler?" asked Marvin.

Yes, it was *the* Dr. Maxwell Andler. The neurosurgeon who had operated on Robert Kennedy, racing unsuccessfully against time after the senator was shot in the Ambassador Hotel. Gene Wyman, Marvin's law partner, had asked this eminent physician to join Drs. Rosin and Brown. Stephanie would have the best doctors available.

"The laboratory facilities are normally closed on Saturdays—but in a situation like this, they'll make an exception," said Dr. Brown. "By tomorrow afternoon we'll know a bit more. At least, what to rule out."

"I believe Stephanie has aseptic meningitis," Dr. Rosin said. "Blood and fluid samples were sent to Atlanta—the Centers for Disease Control—today. We'll know more when they grow the cultures. But it takes six weeks for results, if viruses are involved."

"Six weeks? Surely she'll be home long before then."

"You must be patient," said Dr. Brown, patting my arm.

Saturday, December 12, 1970

Again I followed the gurney and the IV on wheels down long never-ending corridors. The doctors allowed me to sit by Stephanie's side in the semi-dark room when they administered the EEG. Small electrodes were attached to her scalp with a gypsum-like, fast-hardening, white material. The wires led to a machine, connected in turn to stylus markers that mapped the activity of both her right and her left brain on a long scroll of paper. Stephanie rested quietly during this procedure.

Later, Dr. Andler approached me. "There is a lot of swelling in your daughter's brain. We have to relieve the pressure by way of a spinal tap. I have to warn you, no matter how many times we have performed this procedure, certain risks are involved."

"What kind of risks?"

"I don't want to alarm you, but if anything should go wrong, if she should move and the needle slip, there might be damage to the spinal cord. The result would be paralysis from the waist down."

I pressed my eyes shut.

Paralysis.

There was no choice. The pressure on the brain had to be relieved. I forced a smile. "I'm glad she's in your hands, Dr. Andler. I know she'll be all right."

He put his hand on my shoulder, gave it a light squeeze, then closed the door gently behind himself when he left.

Later in the afternoon I sang lullabies to Stephanie as she lay on her fleece-covered bed, apparently asleep.

Marvin entered. "How is my Pumpkin-Face?"

Slowly she opened her eyes, looking first at her father, then searching for me.

I gathered her into my arms. "Hey, Shnooky-Pooh, you're awake—how do you feel?"

Stephanie swiveled her head from Marvin to me, but her stare was blank. She made no sound. The nurse had observed us through the window and entered the room with a 7-Up and a straw. I took the glass from her and propped Stephanie's head up to enable her to drink. She tried to suck on the straw, but the liquid ran down her chin and neck. She was unable to swallow. The nurse brought water. "Try to get some of this down her throat. She needs the liquid."

Then we were called out of the room. Dr. Robert Podosin, a pediatric neurologist had joined the team of doctors. Six of us—four doctors and we, the parents—gathered in the hallway.

Dr. Andler spoke first. "We have ruled out a tumor, an aneurysm, epilepsy or any disease that might have been dormant and that would now begin to affect Stephanie's nervous system. What we have not ruled out, however, is meningitis or encephalitis. It is my opinion that she suffers from the latter." He turned to me, "I believe you told Dr. Brown that her nasal passages were filled with mucous the morning of her convulsions. I believe, as do my colleagues here," he nodded to Drs. Rosin and Brown, "that she suffered an attack during the night." Dr. Andler again addressed me. "Didn't you tell me she complained about vomiting when she woke up?"

"Yes. She said something like, 'Mommy, I threw up.' But I saw no. . .no evidence. . .She did have a lot of mucous, greenish. I wondered about that. It didn't look like from a cold."

"You said she slept in her own room, by herself?"

"Yes, Doctor. Alone."

"Then if she did convulse, no one would have known. The only indication would have been the mucous, later."

I dug in my pocket for a tissue and felt a deep sorrow, imagining Stephanie had been convulsing with no one near to help her.

The doctor paused for a moment, then he put his hand on my shoulder and asked, much like a friend making conversation, "Tell me about your recent trip to Mexico."

I told him we had taken the children out of school for a few additional days after Thanksgiving. We had planned an extended family get-together, including Marvin's parents, the old Judge Finkelstein and his wife, Rosie. We had been in Acapulco many times before, usually in the spring. No one had ever become ill. This time we had chosen the Pierre Marquez Hotel, a few miles outside of Acapulco, for its unpolluted beaches and clear waters. But at the end of the rainy season, driving from the airport to the hotel, we saw cows knee-deep in meadows covered by black water, floating blue hyacinths. I had found the scene bucolic. There were clouds of mosquitoes wafting across the waters, and the horses for hire on the beach looked sickly and tired. We were teasing Stephanie that her blood must be sweeter than ours, since her arms and legs, more than anyone else's in the family, were punctured by mosquito bites.

Dr. Andler listened, scratched his head, nodded.

Later that day, the doctors decided that Stephanie could be transferred from intensive care to a private room.

"If you would like to spend the night with your daughter, we'll have the hospital bring in a cot for you," Dr. Rosin suggested. "That would probably be good for Stephanie's outlook, now that she's conscious."

I smiled a thank you. It felt as if the thunderstorm was slowly passing.

A little while later on my cot, I heard a small voice say, "Mommy?"

"Yes, Steffi, I'm here. I'm right here with you." Soon I was comforted and lulled to sleep by the sound of my child's rhythmic breathing.

Sunday, December 13

The Venetian blinds made the sun paint golden stripes onto the ceiling, awakening me to a brilliant California day. When I raised my head I saw Stephanie sitting up in bed. An immense weight lifted off my chest. I could breathe again. My mood changed to bright, like the sun playing with the soft green walls and the window blinds. A nurse entered, pushing the tray-trolley with breakfast to Stephanie's bed. She was awake by now and looked at the food, at the nurse, and at me. A shiny Stephanie-smile spread across her face, infectious, making the nurse and me smile back.

"Hi, Mom." By this time I had reached her bed and was hugging her. Feeling her close like this, and conscious, was like a tonic of warm milk and honey to my raw nerves.

"I like the butterflies on your hat," Stephanie said as she pointed to the cornflakes on her plate.

"The butterflies on my hat?"

"Hmm. The macaroni on your blouse. . .there!"

Chapter Three

Chrysalis

Later, Sunday morning

Stephanie was conscious now and no longer convulsing. But I had left her "eating butterflies from my hat." Had her brain been damaged by her seizures? I had little knowledge of the workings of the mind, and terms like *aphasia*, when a stricken person thinks of a particular word but cannot speak the word and says something completely different, those terms and conditions were not known to me. I was still confident that Stephanie would be home for Christmas.

However, I felt uneasy as I drove home. I had driven this route a myriad of times, but for some reason I felt more acutely aware of every turn in the road, of every building as Sunset Strip turned into Sunset Boulevard. The tree-lined avenue, with its large stone mansions told tales of an earlier time when Hollywood was young and fortunes were made from dreams on celluloid and translated into dreams of stone.

The landmark pink bungalows of the Beverly Hills Hotel appeared, as they still do on postcards, framed by bottle-green paper cut-outs of palm trees. We had made reservations there for the annual Christmas lunch. It was a highlight of the holiday season the children looked forward to.

My thoughts tumbled as I turned north at the corner of Benedict Canyon and Sunset and then headed west to our secluded street. Seeing our home appear when I turned the corner made me feel warm and safe. The two-story Tudor-style house was a California fantasy of Chester or Oxford, but with Stephanie in the hospital I would gladly have made a Faustian bargain—with angel or devil—and traded this lovely house for the smallest hovel if only Stephanie would be made well.

This house on Ridgedale Drive sheltered our family like a breathing, protective presence. This was the first house I could call my own, and a grand first house it was. But sometimes I woke from a nightmare. I dreamt I wasn't married at all, and my life was an illusion. I found myself back amid the bombed-out ruins of postwar Berlin. In the dark, and only half-awake, I glanced at the shadow of my sleeping husband, and hearing his gentle snore, I slipped back into my own slumber. No, I had not dreamt this life. I was the same immigrant who had arrived eighteen years earlier with a debt to Mormon relatives of five hundred dollars for my passage. I was indeed married to the man I had fallen in love with at first sight, just like in a romance novel, a man both good-looking and highly intelligent. It was hard for me to believe this man loved me back.

Life seemed perfect, but then something seemed to be missing—yes, a baby. After extensive examinations, the doctors told Marvin that he had no sperm. None. He would never father children. A private adoption service arranged the details, and soon we became the parents of Steven, then two weeks old.

But miracles do happen, and I conceived. Marvin had been in Freudian therapy for several years, and the good doctor (Joseph Teicher, MD, professor at USC) took credit for this miracle when he published an article in a psychiatry journal on how he helped a patient's psyche (Marvin Finell's) achieve a breakthrough and develop sperm, overcoming his formerly self-imposed sterility. This seemed strange to me—that he, the doctor, enabled Marvin to create this wonder that grew inside of me. I thought the doctor's theory was ludicrous. For the first time in Marvin's life, he felt a genuine desire to have a family, a desire he had not experienced in his previous marriage. It was Marvin, with a little help from me, who had created this baby. Nine months after Steven became ours, Stephanie was born. We named her for her brother, whom I thought would almost be a twin to her.

I lived the California dream and was fully aware of my good fortune. But I have to admit, our lives had their degree of superficiality. Cocktail parties, charity balls, horse races, trivial pursuits. Still not all was frolic and frou-frou in my life. I was working toward a doctorate in English literature at the University of California at Los Angeles, often studying until the library closed at 2:00 a.m., then getting up a few hours later to get the children ready for school.

Our ordinary lives came to an abrupt halt when Stephanie entered the hospital.

"Anybody home?" I cried out when I entered the house through the back door. I walked through the kitchen just as Celia rushed from her room. Her concern was *Estefani*. I told her, she ate solid food and I expected her home for Christmas. A big smile stretched Celia's wide lips even wider.

I gave her a hug. "Where's Steven?"

"Oh, he next door. Play with Mark."

At the neighbors' Steven flew into my arms. "Mommy, Mommy!" His brown hair looked more tousled than usual. His head reached above my waist as he clung close. "Are you staying home now, Mom?"

"No, honey, let's have lunch. Then I have to go back. I only came home to give you a hug."

"Oh." His voice dropped. "Can't I come with you?"

I hesitated for a moment. Then I thought, *Why not?* "OK, then. But you know you'll have to wait in the lobby. You're not allowed in the children's wing."

"I'm a child."

"Rules. Stupid hospital rules. Maybe the Rothmans will be there, that would be good. You could be with Robyn and Susie."

We arrived in the main vestibule of the hospital at 4:30 p.m. I looked for Frank, Marvin's third law partner, but only found Lorraine, his wife, and their two young daughters seated on the shiny upholstery of the plastic sofa, leafing through magazines.

Lorie waved me a hello. "Frank's in with Steff. He's been gone for quite a while," she said, consulting her watch. "Quite a while." Lorraine pulled a few dollars from her wallet and handed them to Robyn, the elder daughter. "Hi, Stevie! Why don't you kids go to the cafeteria and get something to drink?" She paused, then went on, "The doctors didn't want us in Stephanie's room all at once. I'll visit when Frank gets back."

I pushed through the glass double doors and headed for the children's wing, half-running, half-walking, impatient to see Stephanie. A pretty nurse rushed past me, a young doctor run-stepping by her side.

"Dilantin," shouted a voice from far down the corridor. "Quick!"

The intern picked up his pace.

"Sorry," wisecracked the nurse, keeping in step with him, "I only have dry martinis in my locker."

"Wait till that kid grows up," quipped the doctor, his voice overly loud. "It'll take triples to get her high."

What kid were they talking about? I glimpsed Dr. Rosin down the corridor. *They're talking about my seven-year-old child!* I felt myself go numb. Then angry. Very angry. Then scenes from *M.A.S.H.*, the movie, flashed through my mind—and I remembered that flippancy served as a shield, jokes sheltered doctors and nurses from their own emotions.

Another doctor came running, "Somebody get the trachea tube. Fast!"

Dr. Rosin's familiar baritone boomed from the end of the hallway. "Where the hell is he? Get him here on the double! Is he taking his beauty nap?" All this commotion happened simultaneously, while I, still running and out of breath, had nearly reached Stephanie's room. A tall square of a man blocked my way.

"Frank?"

He grabbed both of my shoulders, forced me to turn around. "You'd better not go near there. Come, I've been waiting for you."

Frank steadied me, steering me by the elbow. My feet felt dead, didn't want to obey. At that moment Marvin arrived. He stopped short when he saw the expression on Frank's face. Frank guided us to a bench. "Don't go to her room. Not now."

Young interns raced past, carrying a black tube-like apparatus. I clung to Marvin, shivering.

Frank motioned toward Stephanie's room. "Dr. Andler is in there. Christ—" He shrugged. "I don't know him from Adam. I go in to visit Steff and see this huge hulk of a man jumping on her and hitting her on the chest. By God, with all his might! I thought he's some loony. . .Tried to drag him off. Mistake. Big mistake. The nurses threw me out." Frank pulled a handkerchief from his pocket and blew his nose. "Then I heard them say Stephanie had a cardiac arrest—"

"Her heart?" I jerked, turned to run to Stephanie's room.

Marvin stopped me. Frank went on. "Lucky that Andler was in there with her. He jumped on her, just in time to start her heart again. He's still sitting there, on top of her, giving her mouth to mouth and pumping her chest."

The doctors continued to yell for the anesthesiologist. Dr. Rosin pushed past, oblivious of us, barking, "Get him over here, now! Goddamn it, this is an emergency! Tell him to drop whatever he's doing and get himself over here!"

Frank explained that they needed the anesthesiologist to push the trachea tube down Stephanie's throat and into her lungs. The cardiac arrest prevented the doctors from entering the tube through the neck.

My head spun. I needed to talk to God. I searched for a place where I could be alone. Any place.

I ran to the door marked LADIES and entered one of the small cubicles. My stomach heaved. I didn't know what would come first, throwing up or prayer.

The smell of disinfectant covering the odor of stale urine made my nose quiver. I sneezed. The brown-stained rim of the white porcelain bowl grew into something sinister, ready to devour me, as my face lowered toward it. The hard cold of the white-and-black tiled floor stabbed my knees. Pain rose, tasting bitter. Kneeling, close to the bowl, I spit phlegm. And I prayed.

I spoke to God as I had never done before. I pleaded from the deepest part of my being. *Please let my child live. Nothing else matters. Stephanie has to live. Please. Please, please. . .*

Someone knocked on the door. Then Marvin's voice. "Are you all right in there?"

"Yes."

"I can't hear you. Speak up!"

"I'm all right. I'll be out in a minute."

I splashed cold water on my face. Put on my sunglasses. Then I closed the door behind me and returned to my seat between Marvin and Frank.

We learned that Stephanie had started convulsing around 1:20 p.m. Drs. Rosin and Brown were present, and later, when the convulsions could not be stopped, Dr. Andler was called to assist. Just as he arrived, and after Stephanie had convulsed for three hours straight, her child's heart gave up. Stopped. Dr. Andler revived the heart. Including the anesthesiologist, five doctors had struggled to save our child's life.

Stephanie survived. It was a miracle. She had won the second round in the battle with "her illness," rising before the count of ten, fighting, still.

That night Stephanie was back in intensive care with nurses watching around the clock. An IV dispensed the necessary fluids and medication. Her slender legs and arms were bruised and punctured from intramuscular shots.

I watched her sleep on a mattress of ice underneath an oxygen tent of clear plastic. Her face looked relaxed, her delicate features wore an enigmatic smile, as though she were time-traveling through fairylands. Her long hair curled beside her soft cheeks, reaching below her shoulders. Dr. Greenberg, a handsome young intern, remarked that she looked like a bronze-haired Snow White in her glass coffin.

Snow White and Sleeping Beauty. Yes, we needed a Prince Charming to kiss her with his magic, to awaken her from her dream—to awaken me from my nightmare.

Earlier, after Stephanie's cardiac arrest, Steven went home with the Rothmans. He couldn't understand why everyone acted so upset and why he couldn't go home with us. I'd tried to explain that his sister's heart had stopped beating. He was not yet eight years old, and though he was a bright child, he could not comprehend that she had almost died, that she was sicker now than before. He pulled away from my arms and trudged behind Frank and Lorraine. When he turned, his blue-blue eyes hooked onto mine, staring in a desperate way. And I watched as Robyn—a few years older—gently took his hand and pulled him along.

It was late when we closed the door to Stephanie's room behind us. The hallways were empty and silent once more when I became aware of my mother. She had kept to herself, not wishing to intrude. I spotted her sitting on a hard wooden bench, her shoulders sagging, clutching a handkerchief. Her eyes were puffy and red.

Mother had remained composed throughout this trying situation. When we were bombed in Berlin during the war, she had run back into the flaming house to rescue my teddy bear and a silver teapot. Later, when the Russians conquered Berlin, she had remained calm and knew how to protect us from being raped. Now, again in an emergency, her conduct reminded me of those years long ago, when my grandmother and I were able to depend on her.

We each had come to the hospital in our own car. Mother lived in Santa Monica, and we shared the same route home, at least part of the way. The traffic was light at this late hour, but the evening's rainstorm was brutal.

The sky had been blue and golden in the morning, but in the evening, clouds towered dark and threatening in the neon-lit night. Then torrents of rain flooded the streets. I observed Marvin rolling down his car window at a traffic signal near our turn-off, flagging Mother down. He stuck his head out of the window—within seconds looking as if someone had poured a bucket of water over him—shouting, "Astrid! It's not safe for you to drive all the way to Santa Monica in this weather. Come, spend the night with us."

I didn't remember ever seeing such a night in California. The wind and the rain whipped the trees that lined Sunset Boulevard, bending them into bizarre shapes. Lightning streaked the sky with ice blue flashes, deafening thunder rolled across the heavens and drowned out traffic noises. When I pulled into our driveway, a black cat leapt in front of my car's headlights and made me jump.

Marvin parked, opened my car door, and noticed my shaking. "It was just a frightened little cat, taking shelter in the garage."

Celia was still awake and offered to make up a bed for Mother.

Every inch of my body ached with fatigue, and yet sleep would not come. When I finally did fall asleep, my overly stimulated brain pulled me into a nightmare whirl of images. Stephanie circled above me, trailing a gown of gauze, her hair reaching far below her waist. A black cat jumped out of the void and grew large, and larger, and bounded after Stephanie. Images of children from the hospital supplanted the cat. Cindy, a girl from Steven's class who lay in a room opposite Stephanie's, appeared with blood spurting from her cancerous jaw. She clutched her chin, then her eyes grew enormously large, and tears the size of golf balls rolled down her cheeks and dropped to the ground. The black cat began to chase the balls made of tears. I looked on in horror as Cindy's chin, her jaw, her mouth dissolved, liquefied, and she grew so huge only her featureless head filled the screen of my dream. I screamed— a silent scream, and while still half-asleep, I saw Stephanie again, her image superimposed on the others, transparent, her long hair glowing bluish-white. I bolted upright in bed. My heart pounded so loud I thought its beat had awakened Marvin, when he took my face in both of his hands, calming me, saying, "She'll be all right, she'll be all right."

It was the thirteenth day of the twelfth month. There was a black cat, thunder, and lightning. I heeded Marvin's reassuring words and dismissed my superstitious thoughts, knowing that whatever evil there was raged in the form of a minuscule virus in our daughter's brain. Little by little, I hoped this evil would be overcome.

Monday, December 14

Another EEG showed little change from the previous one. Stephanie still didn't speak. We were told it would be painful for her now, after the tube had been pushed through her throat close to her vocal cords. The nurses put her on the potty. She said, "I'm done." She did speak! Dr. Andler asked her to pull the pen from his shirt pocket. She moved coherently and was able to make correct responses.

Tuesday, December 15

The doctors put Stephanie on steroids. They performed another spinal tap and inserted an IV to feed her plasma, to help build up her antibodies. The hospital routinely took her blood. I imagined the laboratory to be inhabited by white-clad vampires that administered plasma and then sucked the fresh blood.

Stephanie still wore some of her Acapulco tan, but underneath this thin veneer lay a sickly, greenish cast. Slowly she seemed to fade, to respond less, to withdraw, slipping deeper and deeper into her coma.

She entered a world of her own and dwelled in a place where no one could reach her. There was nothing the doctors could do for her now, but keep her alive with fluids and medication by way of the IV and periodic tapping of her spinal fluid. The steroids were administered to reduce the swelling of the brain. The swollen cerebral matter pressing against the skull would lead to scarring and possible brain damage. Stephanie was kept on the ice blanket, and the oxygen tent still enshrouded her.

Brain fluids. Gray matter. I imagined the formerly peaceful hills and dales of her brain's convolutions besieged by horrific storms—interior storms echoing the weather outside. The brain deluge was wiping out definitions, creating badlands interspersed with puddles of muddy water. Spinal taps kept the waters from rising too high.

Chapter Four

Moments of Light

The alarm shrilled in a high pitch. "Seven o'clock already?" Marvin yawned.

"Yes." I was tempted to pull the covers higher over my head, feeling perpetually tired these days.

"Why don't you sleep a while longer? I'll wake you before I leave," he said.

"I may as well get up too."

A little later, Steven screeched up the stairwell. "Mom! Celia wants me to have oatmeal. I want Cream of Wheat!"

"Just a minute." I rushed downstairs.

Celia had of late been antagonistic toward Steven. Perhaps she resented his being at home while Stephanie was far from her care.

"Steve, hey! Big boy, let me have a look at you. Did you pick out these clothes?"

"Yeah. You like?" He smiled.

"Looks fine. Good combination, shirt, sweater—"

"Yea, yea, yea, I know my colors."

"Now why don't you eat your cereal? The bus will be here in a few minutes."

"I hate it!" he banged on the table. Red shot into his eyes, his innocent smile mutated into the grimace of one of his comic book monsters. "I'm not eating. She knows I hate oatmeal!" he said, pushing the bowl of cereal to the far side of the table.

"I guess then you'll have to go without breakfast. I'm sad, Steven. We're all living under a lot of stress, and you make a fuss about cereal. Why are you giving Celia such a hard time?"

"She! She's not making anything I like. Stephanie, Stephanie. . .that's all she can think of. The *muñequa*. . .His face twisted, showing both anger and repugnance. "The *niña* likes oatmeal. So I get it every morning. Ugh!"

"Tomorrow I'll make you German apple pancakes. Special. But you should eat now, before school. Okay?"

He calmed down, shoveling the by-now-cold oatmeal into his mouth. I reached over the table and stroked his hair.

The horn of the school bus sounded. He grabbed his schoolbag, ran out of the house, and within seconds hopped onto the yellow bus.

I waved goodbye, closed the front door, paused, and leaning against it, felt comforted by the strength of the wood. Then I returned to the kitchen.

"*Señora*, me very nice to Esteban." She was close to crying. "*Señora*, you spoil heem."

"Celia," I said, cutting off any further reproach, "Steven's having a rough time. We must all treat him a bit special during these weeks. He's not even eight, just think! He doesn't understand."

The look on her face told me that *she* didn't understand either. She felt reprimanded. We all were touchy. All I wanted was to be left alone and conserve my strength for Stephanie.

Marvin and I met for lunch almost daily at the Bantam Cock on La Cienega, midpoint between the hospital and Marvin's office. During my absence from the hospital, Mother took my place at Stephanie's bedside. On my way back to the hospital, I passed Blessed Sacrament, a Catholic church, on Sunset Boulevard.

I was raised Lutheran but felt both warmth and comfort in Catholic churches. The mystery of the darkened nave and the spice-sweet scent of incense opened my heart. Of late though, the glimmer of the innumerable votive candles had taken on a different meaning for me. I saw them as flickering lives. Lives in peril.

I would light a seven-day candle in a side chapel. Here I knelt before a mosaic of Christ floating on a cloud, pointing to his own red and open heart. The candles' glow—moving lights and shadows—breathed life into the mosaic. In those moments, Christ on the wall entered me, and He spoke to me as I spoke to Him. I don't remember the words, it was spirit talk, or a dream with floating images conveying meaning. But I felt calm when I left the church, and I felt assured that He loved my child.

Back at the hospital, I hugged Mother and took her place next to Stephanie's bed. I love the classics—Shakespeare, Donne, and Blake—yet I couldn't read any of my favorite poets during this period. The only book I could focus on was the Bible. This struck me as strange since I was not a religious person in a formal sense. I opened pages at random. The Old Testament, the New, the Psalms, the Sermon on the Mount, the Book of Job—yes, especially the Book of Job.

One afternoon, when I returned to the hospital after my mother had already left, I quietly opened the door to Stephanie's room. There she lay, her long hair fanning out on the pillow in bronzed waves. Asleep, as always, asleep.

But behind her, against the light green wall, I noticed something else, a bright and luminous light. Something spread out from it, enfolding Stephanie's head. I stared. And slowly, as I stared intensely at this apparition, the strange shape seemed to draw within itself. It dissolved. Disappeared. I was left gazing at the blank wall, the same shade of light green it had always been.

Chapter Five

The Devil's Choice

Minutes, hours, then days slipped by until I lost all sense of time. Time became an abstraction, it would bend and reel forward then spool back again. I spent my days with Stephanie—from early morning until late at night. I gazed at her, seeming so peacefully asleep, and I would conjure up the dancing Stephanie, in her ballet class, who had out-danced so many of her co-students, Stephanie in a pink tutu, gracefully bending her arm over her head at the ballet barre. Then in my mind I saw her changing, like in a family movie, from a little ballerina in dance class to my rambunctious Stephanie, running full speed toward me when I picked her up from Brownie meetings, falling into my arms, out of breath, hugging me hard. Graceful Stephanie, always in motion, with her hair flying and full of energy. And now she lay motionless in a coma. It was impossible to comprehend.

Marvin came at various hours as his law practice allowed. He never stayed long; he couldn't bear to see his daughter comatose.

"You stay with her," he'd say. "There's nothing I can do. Nothing. . .No, no, you handle it." The rhythm of his leather heels could be heard through the windows of Stephanie's room, as they paced a clickety-clack beat outside. He was never without the brown stub of a cigar clenched tightly between his teeth. Back and forth he paced, chewing, puffing.

Late in the afternoon we left in our separate cars, Marvin to go back to the office, I to go home and prepare dinner and spend time with Steven.

Stephanie's illness became an increasing mystery to her brother, and the hospital rules created a gulf between brother and sister. I didn't understand the reason that siblings under fourteen were not allowed to visit the children's wing. It seemed unjust, especially since there were no communicable diseases involved. It was only natural that a brother would be curious about his sister and the other children I had spoken about in the hospital.

In the room opposite Stephanie's lay Cindy, the girl I had dreamt of, a girl Steven knew from school. She had a malignant tumor removed from her jaw.

"How's Cindy?" Steven asked. "Does she play with Steff?"

"No, Steven. I told you. Stephanie is lying on an ice blanket, with tubes connected to her. She's in a coma. That's like being asleep. She can't play."

"Well, it's time for her to wake up. She'll like Cindy when she does. She's neat."

"It looks like Cindy's going home."

"Bet she's happy. Just before Christmas."

"Yes." I drew him near. "Yes, her parents are lucky. They'll all be together for Christmas."

Steven could not comprehend the reality behind the word *coma,* nor why his sister continued to lie on an ice blanket in an oxygen tent, seemingly asleep.

"Is she sort of dead then?" he asked.

When he mentioned the word *dead*, I lost focus. I stammered when I tried to explain. "No, Steven, she is. . .like. . .One day soon, she'll wake up. And one day she'll be well." I heard my voice rise with an artificial cheerfulness. My fingers ran through his thick hair. "Stevie, we have to be patient. I love you very much, but Stephanie needs me more now. Please, try to understand why I spend so much time with her."

"Mom, if she's asleep, she won't know if you're there or not. So why don't you. . .Want to play checkers?"

We played. I couldn't concentrate. He won.

I tried to be an attentive mother to him, but children know. Steven sensed my wandering thoughts, and he heard the undertones in my voice that gave away the lie of my spoken words. Steven sensed my impatience to rush back to the hospital. He said, "You better hurry on up, Mom. See you later alligator. Bye." His small voice trailed off as I ran out the door.

Each night, after dinner, Marvin and I returned to the hospital. Sometimes we took the Coldwater Canyon route, a few miles longer, but saving us—depending on traffic—perhaps ten minutes of driving time. We zigzagged in serpentines over the hills that separate the Los Angeles basin from the San Fernando Valley. My concern for Stephanie made me blind to the view I used to love—the city stretching on without limits, without borders, strewn with millions of glittering emeralds, rubies, and diamonds, laid out in neat squares in the carpet of night, while the many swimming pools gleamed like polished pieces of turquoise from a Navajo's belt. And through the radiance of this "City of Light" snaked the Ventura Freeway. Then we reached the Hollywood Freeway, and Cedars of Lebanon Hospital on Fountain Avenue was not far.

But for Stephanie, nothing ever changed.

Flowers and holiday arrangements invaded her room and overflowed into the hallway. Toys with garish neon-colored balloon attachments floated into view. I was amazed at how my perceptions had changed. In prior times I would have enjoyed these holiday arrangements. One particular evening I found a large Christmas wreath with a lacquer-red satin ribbon at the foot of Stephanie's bed.

"Take that thing out of here. Now!" I shouted. The nurse looked at me with a puzzled expression. I apologized for my outburst and explained it reminded me of funerals. I knew my behavior was irrational. Clients and business partners, people who didn't know Stephanie, sent gifts. Expensive sets of books arrived. Books on ballet, collections of fairy tales.

"Why don't they send some books of airplanes and trains that I could read, Mom?" Steven asked, eyeing the books I brought home. "Don't they know she's asleep?"

"Let's hope Steffi will come home soon. You know she loves her ballet class. She'll appreciate these books later." That afternoon I went to Dutton's and bought him books on airplanes, telling Steven they were gifts from clients, just for him.

Christmas was but a few days away. I don't remember how or when we decorated the tall tree we bought the night before Stephanie began convulsing. My favorite time of year had turned into a time of utmost despair. I baked no German Christmas *Stollen,* no cinnamon stars. Had it not been for Steven, there would have been no semblance of Christmas at all.

Celia went quietly about her chores, a helping shadow. She loved Stephanie with a fierce devotion. A seven-day votive candle flickered in her bathroom. When I asked her about it, she told me that she had made a vow. She would light a candle every week for the rest of her life if *EL SEÑOR* would let *her* Stephanie live.

Dr. Sidney Rosin, in the uniform of his blue-gray sharkskin suit, stopped Marvin and me in the hallway leading to Stephanie's room. Many of the tests were confirmed by now. I asked about Stephanie's condition. "And her heart, is it all right after the cardiac arrest?"

"Yes, her heartbeat is regular," he answered. "There seems to have been no damage. Her lungs are all right. Kidneys, liver, all are working properly."

"Thank God," Marvin and I said as one. I added, "Great. Then there was no damage done to her vital organs."

"Mrs. Finell," Dr. Rosin's voice dropped. He gently placed a hand on my shoulder, "Her brain is affected. The brain is the most important organ of them all."

It took a moment for his statement to sink into *my* brain. I had thought all along that, after a few more days, Stephanie would wake up from her sleep and all would be as before. *The brain is the most important organ of them all.* The words spun round and round, whirling in circles in my head, even though, at that time, I did not grasp the devastating totality of the truth the doctor tried to tell me.

He continued. "I believe she has encephalitis. In fact, I'm sure of it. Of all the various types, equine or herpes are the ones in question. Of those two, herpes can be treated. Tell me again, you took her water skiing in Acapulco?"

"Yes. She caught on quickly. She was rather good at it." Marvin smiled with a touch of parental pride.

"Did she take any tough spills where the water was forced up her nose?"

"Well. . .yes. In the beginning." I paused. I stared at the doctor. What did he mean? Was the herpes virus active in the bay of Acapulco? "Doctor, how could it get from her nose into her brain?"

"At her age the membranes are very thin. It's just possible that water, carrying the virus, was forced up the nasal passages. It could permeate the membranes, break through the blood-brain barrier. That's what I'm trying to figure out. Could that have happened?" Dr. Rosin looked at me, then at Marvin. His chin touched his chest. His steel-framed glasses slid down his nose when he looked up. "Did you ski in the bay itself?"

"Yes. We crossed the bay on skis several times. From the point beneath the rocks, the Caleta, to the Hilton Hotel. You know, where people parasail."

"Hmm." Dr. Rosin scratched his head. "At the Caleta. . .that's where they run untreated sewage into the bay." He seemed to be familiar with the area. "Very polluted water. All kinds of things afloat there. Hepatitis, herpes—" He looked at me. "Did she have any fever blisters following your trip?"

I shook my head, *No.*

Dr. Rosin continued. "Now, listen carefully. What I'm going to tell you is serious." He took a deep breath and held it for an unusually long time. "There is a serum available; we can obtain this. A doctor in Chicago discovered it. The problem is it only works on the herpes virus. We could use it on Stephanie. However, one-third of the patients. . .Well—" He stabbed the floor with his ice-gray eyes, his fingers twisting his globolous earlobe. "On some it won't work." He shifted his focus, now staring at us, jabbing in our direction with his right index finger. "But there is the chance, a 66 percent chance, that the injections will work."

"The alternative? What's the alternative? What happens to the other 34 percent?" I heard my voice cracking. I stared at him. He stared at me. I felt as if he were paralyzing me.

"Death?" I whispered.

"Yes." He said it quietly but quickly added, "However, the serum works fast, where applicable. The virus is killed and the swelling in the brain goes down. It greatly diminishes the risk of severe brain damage. We have to act quickly. Before more damage is done." He put his hand lightly on my shoulder. "I know it's a tough choice."

I panicked. "But Dr. Rosin, you said she might have equine encephalitis? Isn't that what you said? What would happen if you inject her with this particular serum and she has the horse-sleeping-sickness?"

He shook his head. His hands clasped behind his back. "Then," his voice trailed off, "she would not survive." He gulped a deep breath. "But, I believe, she has the herpes virus. If that is the case she would have a 66 percent chance with this serum. Think," he jabbed his index finger at me again, "the serum kills the virus quickly. I must repeat: the swelling goes down and Stephanie comes out of the coma with minimal brain damage."

The doctors knew the history of our trip. Because of the children, we had stayed far from the bay and crowded downtown Acapulco. All of us loved the beach at the Pierre Marquez hotel, wide and clean, washed by turquoise waters. And there were horses to ride. How could such an evil as encephalitis lurk within this innocent beauty?

Venezuelan equine encephalitis was the only other likely strain of virus causing Stephanie's illness. It originated in South America, jumped the Panama Canal and made its way north, transmitted by its vector: blood-sucking mosquitoes.

What if the equine virus had invaded our daughter's brain? The cultures would take more than another thirty days to grow and only then give us specific results.

But Dr. Rosin spoke of a possible cure. He believed it was the herpes virus infecting her, since textbooks stated that with the equine virus adult humans had a survival rate of only 5 percent. Seven-year-old Stephanie was beating the odds by virtue of still being alive. The conclusion that the virus was the milder herpes virus seemed logical to the doctor.

A cure existed. *If* she suffered from herpes. If not, *the cure would kill.*

My instincts told me Stephanie had contracted the horse sleeping-sickness. We had not water-skied that often. Mosquito bites had covered her arms and legs with hundreds of small red welts.

My eyes again met those of Dr. Rosin. Marvin and I looked at each other. No words were spoken, seconds ticked away. Our eyes agreed. Our shared answer to Dr. Rosin was NO.

That night I heard "Oh Little Town of Bethlehem" sung by sweet-voiced high school carolers strolling down the hallway with their fresh faces, bearing gifts for the hospitalized children. For Stephanie, they left a blond woolly bear. I smiled, this was so right. The bear is a symbol of Berlin, the city I came from, as it is of California, Stephanie's native state. *This little bear will bring her luck.* I felt a moment of hope when I placed it next to Stephanie's shoulder underneath the oxygen tent.

Then, an enormous sadness overwhelmed me. I ran from the room. Down the hallway and back into my cubbyhole of a toilet. A slick paper toilet-seat cover served as a gag to muffle my sobs.

Driving home in the rain, I broke down. Marvin pulled the car over and pulled me into his arms. "She'll be all right. You'll see. She'll be fine. Don't give up hope." He stroked my hair. "I tell you, she'll be all right." He fell silent for a while, then he went on, "We made the right decision. Just think if the serum hadn't worked, how we would feel? Killing our own child. Damn this devil's choice. . .She'll get well." He repeated the words over and over until I stopped crying.

I prayed a lot those days, but comfort escaped me. I tried to conjure up the memory of the "luminous" shape I had seen behind Stephanie's bed. Was that not a sign that she was protected? Then came doubts again. Maybe I had imagined it, my eyes had played tricks. There were moments when I felt intense despair, sensed that my child was slipping away. Suddenly something in the room would feel different. Her heart monitor had not changed its green spikes, but somehow she seemed to be diminishing.

In those moments I took Stephanie's hand into mine and talked to her, believing she could hear me. "Stephanie," I'd whisper, "I love you. I've waited so long for you to come into my life. Please, Stephanie, gather your strength. Stay. Stay with me, stay with your daddy. Please, Stephanie. Stay here, don't go. Please, Steffi, please."

There were times when I could feel life flow like a current between her hands and mine. Nothing external changed. Yet there something intangible passed between her body and my own. *I will not let you slip away, Stephanie. You have to live.*

We made a pitiful attempt to create something resembling a Christmas spirit in the hospital room. I decorated it with a few German *Rauschgold Engel*—wax angels adorned with large golden wings—and boughs of sweet-smelling pine. Mother placed a platter of German sweets, marzipan, and cookies for visitors and nurses on the night stand.

Christmas came and Christmas went. There was no change with Stephanie.

Marvin's parents arrived a few days after the holidays. We had notified them of their grandchild's illness while they were on a cruise in the Caribbean.

They'd stopped for a change of clothes in Chattanooga, Marvin's hometown, and took the next flight to Los Angeles. At the airport Rosie, or Gammy (Marvin's mother), wept when she saw us. "How is our Stephanie?" she whispered when we embraced.

"Is she better, is she out of the coma?" Poppy asked.

"No," I shook my head.

We drove straight to the hospital. Gammy remembered another ride from the airport with the same destination, a little more than seven years earlier when I lay at Cedars giving birth to Stephanie. Marvin had phoned his mother when I went into labor early, on a November Sunday. She boarded the first available flight and arrived that same evening in time for Stephanie's birth.

So many memories connected Rose to our children. She was visiting with us when Steven came into our life. We had just returned from a trip to San Francisco with Rose and were having cocktails in the living room before dinner. The telephone rang. It was Sol Grayson, Marvin's friend and former law partner.

"Sol? What?" I didn't understand. "Me, a mother? Tomorrow morning?" Sol went on talking while Marvin snatched the receiver from my hand.

Rose gave me a bewildered look. "Imagine!" I explained to her. "You remember the baby we wanted to adopt? Yes, the one where the mother changed her mind? Sol just now told me that she gave birth to a healthy baby boy. It seems she can't keep him. I can't believe it! We'll be parents tomorrow morning!"

When Marvin and I embraced that night, it felt different somehow. *I am going to be a mother*, I thought. I felt a deep joy, different from sensual pleasure. *I am going to be a mother; I'm going to be a mother*. The thought kept playing through my mind like a stuck gramophone record.

Little did I imagine that I was going to be a mother *twice*. Stephanie was born nine months later, to the day.

Those nine months were among the happiest in my life. Forget the morning sickness, the throwing up. Beyond this inconvenience I carried a happiness within me that seemed to be visible to all. Even with a growing belly, I was told I'd never looked this good, this radiant. Then, after about four months, I felt the first quiver. As if I had swallowed butterflies. Perhaps *that was* the one most perfect moment in my life: I held my belly, tried to contain this faint flutter within the palm of my hand. It was such a miracle to feel those strange stirrings in my body, of my body yet independent from my body. Knowing that a tiny human being was growing inside of me I experienced a bliss I never could have imagined before. I lay down and turned onto my stomach, then the faint movements would grow more intense. When Marvin came home, I greeted him with a smile he later called "Karin's secret-joy smile." When he placed his hands on my belly, the quiver grew stronger, as if the baby were pleased by the attention. His lips moved between a grin and a smile, and a glow spread over his face as his hands felt the new life growing.

Steven too brought me much happiness during those days, radiating a blue-eyed smile when I rushed home between classes at UCLA to hold him and feed him his bottle. In the classroom, as my abdomen grew, I would at times burst out in laughter. This was embarrassing. I could not tell my fellow students, years younger than me, that my baby's flutters had suddenly grown into jolts and kicks, that odd angles of knees and elbows punched me from the inside. They might have thought me crazy if I had told them these kicks felt delicious.

Now, driving to the hospital, Rose spoke of her own memories. She spoke of the first time she saw her new granddaughter. Nine and a half pounds of baby girl, naked, still covered with birth fluids, lying next to me on the gurney. At last a child had been born to the son she had thought sterile. Marvin, the son she adored, had produced a miracle for her as well. Rose Finkelstein had thought she would never forgive her son for marrying a gentile—a *shiksa*—and then fell unconditionally in love with an animated bundle of not quite ten pounds of flesh, this baby, who smiled from the moment of her birth—the nurses told us this was highly unusual—at a world that was to hold such sorrow for her, and Stephanie became our bond.

A New Year had begun. The presence of Marvin's parents and the attention they gave to Steven improved our son's mood, but Stephanie's situation didn't change. She remained asleep. Cindy, the little girl whose parents I envied when she went home for Christmas, was back in the hospital. The cancer had spread. More of her jaw was removed. A few days later she died, leaving me with a terrible mix of emotions: shame for my former envy, compassion and a deep sadness for her short life and for her grieving parents, as well as gratitude for Stephanie's being alive.

One night Marvin gazed at Stephanie for a long time, and I noticed an increased desperation in him.

We drove home in a hard rain. In the house, Marvin flung his suit jacket onto the couch, ripped off his tie, opened the French doors leading from the family room to the terrace. He stepped out into this weather, leaving the doors wide open. I followed him as far as the doorway, shaking my head.

He stood illuminated in a band of light, as if on stage. I noticed the throbbing veins in his neck when his face turned toward the thundering sky and his rugged features twisted into the grimace of a gargoyle. Water streamed down his face, plastering strands of hair to his forehead.

Then he screamed. "I hate you, God!" Clenching and shaking his fists at the Invisible in the sky.

"I hate you, son-of-a-bitch-fucking God!" And again, and again, falling onto his knees, sobbing, pounding his chest, "Do it to me! *Not to her.* Do it to *me!*"

Slowly he rose, still shaking his fists. Then he crumbled onto his knees again, his arms cradling his head, rocking, touching the terrace stones. The heavens kept on raining. No thunderbolt struck him down to prove: *Yes, I, the God you profess to hate, do exist.*

I went to him, put my arms around him, and led him back into the house. I half-dragged him upstairs and ran a hot bath. Marvin seemed numb and needed help climbing into the tub. I lit candles and told him all the things we would do once Stephanie was well again. He loved it when I sang to him. In the steamy bath I began, "Es la historia de un amor, que no hay otra igual, que mi hizo comprender todo el bien, todo el mal," a song by Augustin Lara we had declared *our* song when we'd first heard it in Acapulco. Why had we selected *that* song? We knew it was written after the death of the composer's wife. A song born out of pain and sadness. This night the words seemed more fitting than during that distant time when all was well. When we first heard it, we danced at the Las Brisas Hotel under a full moon high above the shimmering bay. But even then, these words—proving so prophetic—touched us, words speaking of a love that has no equal, a love that teaches, that makes one understand all that is good and all that is bad. Todo el bien, todo el mal.

Slowly, with my singing, Marvin relaxed, a sparkle returned to his Tartar eyes and, on impulse, he pulled me into the oversized tub. Clothes and all.

Chapter Six

The Awakening

Six weeks had gone by, and Stephanie still lay in her coma. It was the twenty-fifth day of January when Dr. Robert Podosin rushed into Stephanie's room, shouting. "The results from Atlanta are back. What a girl! She's alive and she's battling the deadliest of them all. Venezuelan equine encephalitis."

I sank to my knees. *Thank you, God! Thank you, that Marvin and I had followed our instincts and not allowed the herpes vaccine to be administered.*

A day later my friend Betty visited us in the hospital. Stephanie's eyes, half-closed, gazed in the direction of the television above her bed. The doctors thought it a good idea to keep the TV on, tuned to shows she'd liked. *I Love Lucy* was playing.

"Ricky," wailed Lucy's voice. "Ricky you must believe me, there was a burglar, yes there was—"

Stephanie suddenly opened her eyes wide and looking at the screen shouted, "Lucy!" She repeated, "Lucy!" Then she said, "No!"

"Stephanie!" I grabbed her to my chest, hugged her, and covered her face with kisses, bathing her face in tears of happiness. Then I cranked up her bed so she could watch the show better.

"Stephanie, you're awake! Oh, I love you, I love you to pieces!"

Betty called the nurse. I grabbed the phone. Dialed. "Marv? Yes, it's me. I can hardly talk. She said 'Lucy' and 'No.' Stephanie. . .yes, of course I'm talking about Stephanie. She's out of the coma! She recognized me. Yes, come. Quick."

But Stephanie was far from well. Those words were all she would say. She still couldn't eat. By now she had progressed from the IV to feeding by tube. She came to hate some foods from that time on, especially carrots and liver, which the hospital fed her in proportionately large amounts. The oxygen tent had been removed some time earlier. The IV was still attached to her ankle to administer medications. We were fortunate that our health insurance allowed us to hire three private nurses who attended Stephanie around the clock.

She could not go to the toilet, nor was she able to ring for the nurse to help her. Soon the feeding tube was removed, and she progressed to eating solid foods and drinking fluids. She needed to be toilet trained. To no avail. The hospital put her in diapers. I wanted to take her home, thinking her progress might speed up within familiar surroundings. The doctors disagreed. Finally, Marvin and I promised the medical staff we would retain the around-the-clock shift of three nurses in our home, for however long they were needed. After much arguing, the doctors allowed us to take our daughter home.

Stephanie had been in the hospital for over seven weeks, six of them in a coma.

It was such a different ride home, Stephanie again sat on my lap, but this time her body was no longer a leaden weight, and she was conscious. Gone was her Acapulco tan. She looked different somehow, so pale, and removed as if she were a stranger to this planet. Only her hair fell in glossy waves as before.

Marvin pulled into the driveway. Steven and Celia rushed out from the back door to greet Stephanie. There was hardly a nod of recognition on Steff's part. Her favorite dog, Kelly, one of our two Westies, ran toward her with her tail wagging to sniff her. She ignored the little dog.

Miss Nunan, the younger one of the three nurses, had followed in her car and entered the house. I caught her eyes evaluating Stephanie's homecoming.

Staggering like a somnambulist, Stephanie crossed the living room to the music room and sat down at the Steinway baby grand. She lifted the cover from the keyboard and began to play "Für Elise," a short and easy piece by Beethoven. I was amazed at how well she still played.

This puzzled me. Stephanie did not recognize her brother, or the dogs, but she knew where the music room was and sat at the piano to play.

Celia brought a tray with lunch, tempting her to eat her favorite—*quesadillas* —but Stephanie pushed the food away. I believed she was overly stimulated and tired, and I coaxed her upstairs to her room.

She followed me, and then she stumbled and fell.

"She's very weak," Miss Nunan said, bringing in a child's walker. "Try her on this, till she gets the hang of walking again."

"Over my dead body," Marvin growled and grabbed the walker and flung it across the hallway. "My daughter is not going to be an invalid. She's going to walk on her own, or crawl until she does. No walker."

Miss Nunan, a large woman, grew red in the face, and I sensed she wanted to reprimand Marvin, or perhaps punch him, but she restrained herself and only raised her eyebrows. She and I looked at each other and kept silent.

Stephanie had reached the stairs, held on to the spindles of the banister, pulling herself up, with Marvin and me following close to catch her if she fell. She made it to the landing. Here she had to turn right, climb another four steps, and walk in a direct line to her room. But instead she turned left. She moved as if in slow motion. Now she faced the leaded glass window on the landing, where she seemed to lose herself gazing at the blown glass sails of an ancient schooner. Then her eyes caught my worried look, and she began her descent.

"Honey, you have to turn right to go to your room," Marvin pleaded, pushing her gently to go up. Again she climbed the stairs. On the landing she made the effort to turn right. Impossible. Her eyes were vacant as she turned left and came down once more.

Finally we took her by the shoulders and walked with her, guiding her to maneuver the "right" turn. When she reached the hallway leading to her room, she jerked herself free of our help and, with arms flailing like a football coach giving signals, indicated she wanted to walk by herself. And she did.

Her eyes brightened the moment she passed the threshold to her room. She smiled back at us, her eyes sparkling as in former times, and I knew we had done the right thing in bringing her home. Stephanie recognized her room. I saw she was happy to be in her familiar surroundings again. With her arms outstretched, she turned in a circle, pointing to the blue-and-turquoise flowered wallpaper. She pointed to the full-sized bed with its Mexican headboard of turquoise-and-lilac papier-mâché kissing doves perched above a heart, and she headed for her bed.

The comforter with its white lace-edged sheet had been turned down, all in readiness for our Stephanie. I pulled off her robe, and she crawled between the sheets, hugging the five-foot Snoopy her uncle Bud had sent her for Christmas a year ago.

During the next few weeks her progress was minute, but steady. We took her to an eminent pediatric neurologist at a nearby university hospital for a second opinion and a complete medical evaluation.

"Vell, when did she go into ze coma? And how long was she in ze coma?"

I asked him if he came from Berlin (his family name was a common name in my city), feeling comforted that my daughter was being seen by a *landsman*.

"I have no *tcherman* accent," he replied emphatically. Then he went on with his thorough examination. In the end, he asked Marvin and me to step into his office.

"What she does not regain in six months, she will not regain. You will know in that time span what hope there is for recovery. You can expect her to throw tantrums, to become very disturbed, very angry."

Sunny Stephanie, throwing tantrums?

He went on, "She will have headaches. Her friends will drop away."

I wanted to run from this prophet of doom. Stephanie had been one of the most popular girls in her class. Her friends were numerous. She would lose them?

He continued, "Her right arm will be paralyzed. She will try to ignore this arm. Make her use it. To prevent her from developing epilepsy, she must go on Dilantin. If there is no progress in six months, you might check into the possibility of an institution for her."

We left. I don't remember saying goodbye.

The doctor's prognosis concerning paralysis in Stephanie's right arm and hand proved correct. She played the piano when she first came home from the hospital, but later she lost the use of that hand. Rather, she carried her right hand aloft, like a communist worker waving his fist.

What had happened was that on her first day home, brain impulses were still transmitted to her right hand. And part of her memory-responses recalled the Beethoven piece, enabling her to sit down and play "Für Elise." What must have been only minutes later, some of the circuits were interrupted and barred the transmission of impulses from one nerve ending to another. Her right hand grew stiff and eventually became paralyzed. Just as the "doomdoctor" had predicted.

Both hemispheres of the brain had been attacked by the virus, the left side more severely than the right. Stephanie was born right-handed. The left side of the brain governed the body movements on her right side, her ability to reason, her short-term memory, and her spatial orientation. The brain fever damaged her speech center, and she was no longer able to articulate words. We were told that Stephanie had to switch from being right-handed to using her left hand.

I read that the brain is a mass of circuitry, with crucial information flowing from neuron to neuron across microscopic gaps called synapses. I imagined Stephanie's brain as one of the early giant IBM computers that Marvin had visited in the 1960s and described to me. Enormous machines that occupied entire rooms. People who entered these rooms had to wear protective and sterile clothing in order not to contaminate the computer. Now one of these rooms had been broken into by vandals, who then played havoc with the intricate electronic programming. Rough hands grasped delicate wires. They ripped and destroyed. Dirty hands contaminated the sterile environment of the computer.

I spoke with a neurologist recently, and he made another analogy, perhaps more fitting—that of a symphony orchestra. The brain is the organ, and the mind is what produces the thoughts, what the mind brings forth. Or the brain is the orchestra, and the mind produces the music it plays. If something happens to disrupt the balance of the players and their instruments, dissonance is the result. In some cases there would never be enough musicians, each with their particular instrument, to make beautiful music again. But in another scenario, as the brain forms new connections, there would be enough musicians and instruments left to form a chamber orchestra. Or if even more limited, perhaps a quartet could be assembled, and they would still be able to play lovely music, although greatly reduced from the former sound of the full orchestra.

In Stephanie's case, much of the wired programming was still intact, but the synapses leading to the terminals were intermittently disconnected. Stephanie's age was to her advantage. Her brain was still growing, and the plasticity of her young brain allowed new routes to form and new connections to be made. The big question was How much of Stephanie's brain could be "rerouted"? How could her orchestra be reorganized to make music again?

So far her doctors had not recommended any therapy. They felt that Stephanie must first regain her stamina and strength.

I wrote to the Institute for the Achievement of Human Potential in Philadelphia. They called their work "Programming of the Brain." The therapy would involve the three of us traveling to Philadelphia and spending weeks, perhaps months there. Marvin rejected the idea. He believed Stephanie's brain had done so much on its own in the last few weeks it might be better not to interfere. I accused him of thinking of his clients and his law firm first, and not of Stephanie. I never won those arguments. He would hug me and assure me he loved us both very much and would do what was right for us all.

We did not go to Philadelphia, but I studied their manual and followed their advice. The institute stressed the importance of crawling on all fours as a pathway to learning. I remembered the old saying *You have to crawl before you can walk*. In crawling, I read, the motion of having to alternate the leg with the opposite hand helps develop the brain, by forcing messages to cross from the right and left hemispheres of the cortex. I insisted that Stephanie crawl. I invented games to crawl the length of the thirty-foot living room with her. She objected, perhaps feeling this was babyish behavior. She'd rather walk, or run. She'd jump up suddenly and run to the stairs; run up the stairs, then down with me chasing her. When she had exhausted herself and me, she'd come over and put her arms around me as if to say, "I'm sorry." She had shown me she could walk and run at a fast clip. I crawled again urging her to follow my example. No, she shook her head not having the words yet, again and again she shook her head, saying *No*. At that time I hoped for better luck the next day, maybe earlier in the morning before other activities had tired her out.

I tried the same procedure right after breakfast the next day. "Steffi, please, try it. It will help you with your right hand."

She again shook her head. No way. There were tantrums. I insisted on crawling. Finally she crawled. She did not open her right hand but bunched it up and crawled on her fist, dragging her right leg as in a limp. Again this struck me as peculiar, as she did not limp when she walked. No doctor could explain this to us.

It was mid-February. The insurance company had reluctantly paid 80 percent of the hospital cost but no longer wanted to pay their share for the nurses in our home. Marvin—a persistent attorney—argued that he was saving the insurance company money if they paid for the nurses, rather than pay the stiff hospital bills. Battles with the insurance company were added to the concern for Stephanie's recovery. In the end we felt that Stephanie's improvement justified letting two of the nurses go. We kept the day nurse, Miss Nunan.

An occupational therapist came to the house several times a week. Stephanie needed to relearn movement coordination. One of these movements was the simple gesture of putting her thumb into her ear and simultaneously wiggling the fingers of her hand. She repeatedly put her index finger into her ear. And this with her left, her *good* hand. The therapist and I kept pointing to her thumb, holding our own thumbs up. Finally she managed. With her thumb in her ear, she smiled her former *See? I can do it* smile.

It filled me with such sadness to witness that every small gesture we "healthy" people took for granted posed an almost insurmountable obstacle to her.

Sunny and warm days followed the heavy rains of winter. Soon the foothills of the Santa Monica Mountains burst forth in vibrant green. The energy of spring infused me with renewed hope for Stephanie's recovery, hope that grew tall like the spring grasses—and as bright as California's golden poppies.

On many of these pre-summer days, I took Stephanie and Miss Nunan to Zuma beach. Here, swings and slides provided exercise equipment. Running barefoot on the sand and playing in the lapping surf gave Stephanie a renewed sense of freedom. We were lucky that few, if any, children were present. Younger able-bodied children embarrassed her in her often awkward attempts at climbing and moving on the equipment.

It was almost a month since Stephanie left the hospital, and she was still in diapers. This made it difficult to take her to places. She objected vehemently when I once suggested changing her diaper in an empty—public—toilet. Her recognition of her age and her frustration with her present stage of development was acute, making me doubly sad.

She spoke a few words by now, one of them, *titi*, meaning she had to urinate. But often she forgot to let us know and wet her pants. I promised her swimming lessons if she learned to tell us on a regular basis when she had to go. Within a week she let me know, "Mommy, titi." Living proof that a little bribe can help.

Stephanie had learned to swim at Anatole's Swimming School for Tots when she was less than two years old. I opened the once familiar door for her, and entering, she swiveled her head and seemed to recognize the indoor pool, crinkling her nose at the smell of chlorine in the vapor-filled hall. She gave Anatole one of her big and happy grins, seemingly remembering him. Later, she looked comfortable and safe in his strong arms, snuggling against his bear-like chest when he placed her into the water with care.

Cautiously he pushed her head under water. "Now blow Stephanie, blow bubbles."

She understood. Bubbles floated to the surface. Soon Stephanie's face emerged, radiant. Smiling. And voluntarily she ducked below the water again and again.

"Before long we'll have her swimming again," Anatole assured me.

The lessons continued. Soon I noticed Stephanie using her right hand more, and it seemed to become more flexible and cramped up less.

And then there were the "deefficukt" days, as Celia pronounced it. I'd heard her this morning on the phone to my mother, "Oh, *Señora*, Estefani is very *deefficukt* today."

"Why do you let that maid criticize your daughter?" Mother said later.

"What did you call Celia? *That maid?* Sometimes she understands Steffi better than any of us."

"You are crazy. You have lost all sense of. . .of. . .propriety."

I shrugged. Celia was right. These days were difficult. Why add to it another argument with my mother? Tensions. High wires, is that not what acrobats perform on? I desperately tried to keep my balance, walking with caution and arms spread out wide on these wires.

Of late Stephanie was acting high-strung. Her long, curly hair tangled easily. Each morning the endless shouting of, "Ouch, no, no, no, Mommy, no," with interruptions of "titi," which she knew so well would bring moments of respite, all of it was maddening.

This morning had been trying. First the hair, then the socks. She kicked and screamed. Everything became a struggle. I knew this behavior was part of the aftermath of her illness. So far, her vocabulary did not include words for *pain*. But pain she experienced at the lightest touch. This came as a surprise. Before the illness her pain threshold had been high, similar to her father's. Stephanie had never flinched when given an injection, never cried when she fell and skinned her knee. All this changed. Her illness drastically altered the responses of her nerve-endings to contact.

We drove to Anatole's in my car. Mother followed in hers.

Stephanie swam breaststroke the entire length of the sixty-foot pool, underwater. I had been studying my appointment book, and when I looked up, I found her sitting on Anatole's arm.

"Hey, don't you pinch me!" He pointed to his upper arm, saying, "Wow. She pinched me. Hard." Then a look of compassion softened his features. "Hey, Steff, you can pinch me, Hon, but only with your right hand. Agreed?"

Opposite of me sat my mother. She too demanded attention. "Karin, listen to what your Uncle Will writes—" Her voice boomed, amplified by the acoustics of the water-filled hall.

At any other time I would love to hear what my uncle, who had visited with us last week from Germany, had written. But not now. Not here. "Mutti, please, I'm concentrating on Stephanie, on her swimming. You know she likes being watched."

Mother would not be deterred. She rose and came toward me. I stood up as well. We both circled the pool. Then I couldn't stand it and broke out in laughter.

"Why are you laughing?"

"Never mind," I said, hiccupping now, amused by what I thought we must look like. Two weary-looking dogs, "bitches," stalking and circling one another.

Stephanie popped up, splashing. "She's a bit uptight today," Anatole said. "She's not opening her right hand."

"You see," Mother took the cue. "She needs therapy. You haven't done a thing about that now, have you?"

"Yes, I have. Next week we're taking her to Rancho Los Amigos. She'll have a full evaluation."

"Rancho Los Amigos!" Mother's nose pointed to the Plexiglas roof. "That's about as bad as that asylum in Camarillo. You should take her to Loma Linda, the Seventh Day Adventist hospital."

"Oh yes. You attended their services the last few Saturdays, right?"

"Don't be sarcastic. Everyone knows they have the best doctors. This other place, that's just—"

I grew angry, sensing that Stephanie could comprehend much of what was being said. "Mother, please. . .We'll talk about it later. It would help if you'd go home now."

"You're telling me to go? Me, your mother?"

She crinkled the letter into her purse, rose slowly, and sauntered out. Mother! She had gone through four years of nightly air raids in Berlin, working two jobs, totaling twelve hours every day. She was brave, and she endured much. I thought maybe this earlier wartime trauma surfaced now. Her nerves were raw, and she easily lost her self-control. She had always wanted to dominate me, strangle me with her possessiveness, and now this extended to her grandchild. She was not only jealous of my relationship to my child, she was also jealous of Celia, or anyone else who was close to Stephanie's affection.

Helping Stephanie get dressed after that scene proved exhausting. My tension had amplified hers.

When we walked to my car minutes later, it was drizzling. Stephanie looked like Little Red Riding Hood, with the top of her red slicker drawn over her damp hair. Then I spotted Mother, coming toward us from the coffee shop at the corner.

"Karin, I want to say one more thing." She shook her index finger at me. "You've had a lot of bad luck lately. If you don't treat your mother better, you'll have to suffer a lot more in your life! You'll see!"

And like Maleficent, the wicked fairy in *Sleeping Beauty*, she disappeared after casting her spell, leaving me gape-mouthed, breathing in the fumes from her exhaust.

Chapter Seven

Slowly, Too Slowly

The river hears music
Music climbs the ocean waves, listen!
—Stephanie Finell

Sunny, sparkling, smog free days followed. Stephanie's sense of music and rhythm appeared to be unimpaired. Although she still couldn't speak more than a few words, she was able to sing and harmonize. She would hum the melody, and here and there she remembered words to songs she'd sung before. I found that when I sang with her, she could relearn words, much as children do when they learn the alphabet by sing-songing it. Stephanie's right hand and arm continued to improve, allowing for limited movement. I saw her stretch both arms to catch the ball her father tossed to her in our backyard and heard snatches of his voice, "Great, Pumpkin, now catch!"

Watching father and daughter through the lace curtains of the kitchen window gave me a rush of warmth, much like the heat of a German tile stove that greeted me in my youth when I came inside after a winter snowstorm. Sometimes Marvin showed more patience than I could muster. I reminded myself that I was lucky in countless ways. Not only was Marvin helpful, but I also had Celia to look after chores in the big house. I knew that the majority of mothers, many with children more severely disabled than Stephanie, had to manage by themselves. A feeling of shame then arose in me, shame that I was so irritable, shame that my tears flowed so freely at any given moment.

The day of our appointment at Rancho Los Amigos arrived. The impending tests were on my mind. Oversized hopes had built dream castles in my mind. Would they be dashed today, like a wave would wash away a sand castle on the beach?

At Rancho Los Amigos, our car passed through wide gates and rolled past landscaped grounds toward the parking lot. We met friendly and caring health-care workers after entering through "The Friends" gate. The staff had kept our appointment to the minute, which was especially appreciated by Marvin, who watched the minutes and hours by his innate "attorney-clock."

A motherly nurse ushered us into an examining room. On our way we passed a trolley cart filled with tiny bikinis to be worn by the young patients.

"Here, Sweetie, I want you to choose a pretty one for the doctor to examine you in." The nurse held up a polka dot affair in pink. "Isn't this pretty? Or this one?" Stephanie chose a purple one with a teddy bear print. The nurse noticed my look of surprise. "We found kids love to wear these. More fun to go from one examination to another than in a drab hospital gown."

A navy-blue corduroy robe completed the outfit, keeping the patient warm. Every doctor who examined Stephanie showed kindness. There was a pervasive spirit of love throughout Rancho Los Amigos, just as our friend had described it.

The consensus after almost a full day of testing was that "Stephanie, all on her own, has made wonderful progress these last two months. Amazing progress. Nothing can be done for her at this time. It would be best not to interfere with her own recuperative powers. She should return in two months time."

Two months. That's a long time for impatient parents.

A few days later, I promised Stephanie I would take her to the Kantors' after her swimming lesson. Ulrike Kantor had also come from Germany, and we'd been friends for years. They lived in the Malibu colony by the lapping waves of the Pacific. When I mentioned Ulrike, Stephanie's eyes lit up.

Lunch was served on the terrace. The sky was a deep pre-summer blue. The ocean was its large azure mirror. At a cursory glance, Stephanie fit in with the other children.

Ten-year-old Paul Kantor arrived home from school and asked his mother, "Where has she learned all this so fast?"

A child's observation. He had seen Stephanie repeatedly during the last few weeks. Adults also mentioned the progress they observed in Stephanie, but I valued a child's candid remark as more straightforward.

I spotted a ball on the beach about eight feet from us. "Steff, please bring me the ball," I said.

She walked straight to it, picked it up with both hands, and brought it back. Then she took two-year-old Neil for a walk on the sand, using her paralyzed right hand for him to hold. After a while she began building a sand castle. I saw her carefully heap and pat the sand with her left hand, holding the right hand rigid, with her fist balled as a non-essential appendage on her stretched-out arm.

Jon Peters was a neighbor who had married one of my favorite actresses, Lesley Ann Warren, and he was sharing a bottle of wine with us on the terrace. Ulrike, earlier, had told him about Stephanie's illness. He watched as she built her sand castle. On impulse, he jumped from the terrace to the sand and crossed to Stephanie. I could not hear what was being said, but I watched as he talked to her, and she turned her face up eagerly when she answered. Soon he crouched by her side and helped with building the castle. Stephanie's posture changed. She held her left hand behind her back as she tried hard to move sand with her right hand. (This is exactly what therapists later advised, to encourage her to use her weak right hand.) Slowly the castle took shape, and Jon was grinning, encouraging. Stephanie smiled back despite the enormous effort it cost her not to use her left hand. I saw him nod. Did she ask for permission to use both hands? Apparently so. For now she dug into the sand with both her left and her right hand in order to complete the castle.

Not only was this fun for Stephanie, but as I learned later, that feeling small grains of sand stimulates nerve endings, similar to the brushes therapists would use in the future.

Stephanie's happiness was infectious. When I saw her face radiating joy, riding high on Jon's shoulders as they approached the terrace, I too felt happy. And I was proud of her for keeping her balance.

The Kantor children and some adults were playing with a mechanical table-foosball game in the family room. Ulrike's house was always filled with Malibu colony neighbors, movie personalities, musicians. I had not met one person in this house who rejected Stephanie or made me or her feel ill at ease. Not until that day.

A minor talent agent, scraggly bearded, with adolescent pimples on his pasty skin was handling the row of plastic foosball players, hitting the ball to the opposing side. He pushed the handle into Stephanie's hand, encouraging her to play. She failed. But she tried again. And again.

"Come on, you can do it," he tried to motivate her, but Stephanie walked away. "What's with her?" The man's voice shouted, overly loud, "Is she retarded or something?"

Retarded! The word struck me as though someone had thrown a knife at me. I hoped Stephanie had not heard, or understood. I reached for her hand and we left.

Steven stopped bringing friends home. This meant more driving for me, not only to his karate class, his tennis, his Little League practice, but also chauffeuring him to his friends' homes.

"Why don't you have Hendryk come over here? I'll start heating the pool and you can both swim."

"No, Mom. I'd rather go to his house."

"But Stevie, it's not fair. Hendryk doesn't have a pool; he enjoys coming here."

"No. He doesn't like to swim."

"That's crazy Steven, I happen to know that he loves to swim. What about Bobby, or some of your other friends?"

"What about them?"

"They haven't come over lately. Would you like a swim and barbecue party?"

"What would you do with Stephanie?"

"She swims again. She wouldn't bother anyone."

"Yes she would."

"How?"

"It's embarrassing, Mom."

"What's embarrassing?"

"To have a mental retard for a sister. That's what."

Mental retard! That phrase was even more hurtful now, coming from Steven. I tried to explain. "Steven, you know your sister was very ill. She has to learn everything all over. She'll be okay again."

"She'll talk again and everything?" He twisted his mouth in a peculiar fashion while his blue eyes focused on me intently.

"Yes, Steven. And she'll go to school again. She's not retarded. But she does have a lot of relearning to do. Her brain has to be retrained. And, Steven, she needs help. From all of us. Do understand, please? We have to help her."

"But, Mom." He shook his head and pushed at the unruly mass of brown hair falling into his eyes. "She embarrasses me. When she drools, when she stuffs all that food into the right side of her face. . .like a chipmunk."

I shook my head. *Damn the tears.* I had to stop the car. My vision had misted up and I couldn't see the road as I drove my eight-year-old to Hendryk's house.

I was impatient and desperately wanted to know the extent of the damage done to Stephanie's brain, and how long this recovery process would take. One doctor had painted a dismal picture of her future, while other doctors gave us hope but no specifics. Marvin and I fumbled along and grabbed at every suggestion. At that time, in 1971, it was impossible to make an accurate assessment of her brain damage. Many of the procedures and techniques such as MRIs, CT scans, and PET scans available to doctors today had not yet been developed.

One of Stephanie's problems was drooling. Especially when she felt pressured in completing a task, such as using building blocks to help with spatial perceptions. The partial paralysis of her right side extended to her mouth, which was less sensitive on the right. This led to saliva running out of her mouth at times and a reduced ability to feel food still left in the right side of her cheeks.

If Stephanie's drooling repulsed Steven, I reasoned, it would repulse others. We made an appointment with a surgeon who operated on cases such as Stephanie's. After he examined her, he discouraged us from an operation. It would have drawbacks. Her mouth would get dry. She would have to take in a great amount of liquids to compensate for the saliva ducts that would have been set far back into her pharynx. The doctor said the option of an operation would still be open to us if the drooling persisted. It was encouraging to hear his opinion—that Stephanie, within the next few months, might develop some control over her drooling on her own.

Chapter Eight

Fissures

Please Lord, Let me know if I can do
Anything—Anything well
> —Stephanie Finell

Imperceptibly Stephanie's illness changed us. It pointed out the superficiality and transient existence of our lives.

The children lay asleep upstairs; pine logs crackled in the living room fireplace. I had put the guitar next to my chair when I finished playing a Spanish dance. The setting would have been cozy, and Marvin usually felt mellow when I strummed these easy pieces, but this time his expression did not change to relaxed and smiling, rather he slouched in his favorite chair, grimly silent, while he swirled the amber liquid of the J&B, furiously, clinking ice cubes against crystal. He put me on edge, downing his third Scotch. His eyes were fixed on the fire, staring, unblinking. Suddenly he broke the silence, almost shouting as if in self-defense, "I'm leaving the firm. I can't take the squabbles anymore."

"You're what?"

"I don't know. . .It's the only move that will keep me sane."

"You mean you're going to leave. . . leave the firm? The law firm *you* built?"

"Gene and I. They don't need me. Klein made me an offer to work for him—"

"Wait. . . Marv, he's your client. I don't understand—I can't see you working for someone else. You've never had a boss."

"Yes I did. When I carried Charley MacCarthy in a suitcase."

"Come on. You were just out of law-school—"

"Yeah, you're right. What a fool I was, thinking I'd get to practice law for the great Edgar Bergen. All he used me for was to carry that damn dummy onto the plane, train, cars, wherever he was going. I was his valet." He chuckled. "An expensive Harvard valet." He twirled the Scotch in his glass with increasing intensity, studying the bursting soda bubbles. "With Gene Klein it's a different story. He won't—technically speaking—be my boss." He continued in a monologue, as if to convince himself this was the right decision. "He won't interfere. Christ, I've been working for Klein now for the past three years. Almost exclusively for him." He stared at the fire again.

The silence was awkward, with only the popping sounds of exploding resin in pine logs that sounded like gun shots. The cozy fire, drinks in Waterford glasses, the guitar; this tranquil setting belied the tension.

"At National General," he continued, "I wouldn't be bugged by these supercilious young Turks. Labels, show, names, I'm sick of it all. I love running the insurance company. I'm damn good at it. I won't have to waste time with superficial crap." He let out a wounded sigh. "It's getting to me."

"Think it over. Don't do anything rash."

"I'd be getting a ten-year contract. Stock options. We'd do all right."

"Will running the insurance company give you *real* satisfaction?"

"Yes. Definitely!" His face took on a triumphant expression when he explained the details of restructuring the company. His slanted dark eyes had always reminded me of the eyes of Mongolian warriors. These Genghis Khan eyes took on the hard glitter of excitement that I had not seen in a long time. "It's like a big game, and when I see the outcome, the figures that spell success. . . I feel great. Just great. 'Cause I did it!"

"You do what you must," I said, though I felt a dark premonition.

The children were happy when Marvin's sister, Aunt Farol, blew into town just before Easter. Her visits always created great gusts of wind—tornadoes, cyclones, or a hurricane, depending on her mood and length of stay. She was flamboyant and she *sparkled*, as Stephanie would say. She was incredibly funny, entertaining, lovable, and annoying. To the children she was an "Auntie Mame."

She planned for us to accompany her to Jim Nabors's house in Bel Air. She had known Jim from long before he became a famous actor-singer. And she thought the children would have fun coming along.

Farol had told Jim about Stephanie's illness. Years ago, when still a toddler, Stephanie had sat on his lap several times. Now she was her usual happy self, humming and bouncing along the garden path, skipping ahead of Steven, Farol, and me. Jim's secretary, Mary, welcomed us, offering the children candies from a silver bowl. Stephanie asked with her eyes, *may I?*

"Go ahead, Stephanie," I said. Steven had finished his candy and was reaching for a second piece when Stephanie began to cough, choking. Her face turned a deep shade of red, and she looked as if she were going to convulse. I panicked. At the time I didn't know the Heimlich maneuver.

"Oh my Gahd!" Jim said, dashing toward us from the house, grabbing Steff by one ankle while I grabbed the other, turning her upside down. Jim slapped her back. Her face turned purple, then blue. She made a strange gurgling sound. Mary was on the phone, calling the emergency number.

Jim kept repeating, "Oh my Gahd," and slapping her back while Stephanie hung upside down—for what to me seemed like an eternity—when suddenly a small round ball flew through the air, hit the flagstone entryway, and broke into a hundred bits of orange.

We let out a simultaneous swoosh of breath. Then Jim sat her down. Stephanie buried her tear-stained face in my waist. Soon, though, she cheered up when Jim made funny faces and when he went into a song and dance routine, just for her.

A few days passed. Then Marvin entered the kitchen and asked, "Who are all the little baskets for?" He pointed to the table where green shredded tissue paper spilled from yellow baskets into which Stephanie and I had placed sugar bunnies and chocolate eggs.

"They're for the children at Cedars," I said.

"Oh?"

"I plan to take Stephanie there on Easter Sunday and bring some holiday cheer to them. Remember how nice it was for us at Christmas to have the carolers come through and distribute presents?"

"I don't remember that. No, not at all."

"Ah, come on," I said. "Don't you remember the little bear they gave Steff?"

"No. Stephanie won't either; she was still comatose. If you must, you go and distribute your baskets." His jaws clenched. "But I don't want Stephanie to go."

Stephanie swiveled her head in bewilderment from her father to me.

"What's. . .? Why?" I asked.

"We'll discuss it later."

"All right, Marv, we can talk now. Steffi's in bed. I do want to take her to Cedars. It'll be nice for her to play Easter bunny to the other children."

"You'll do no such thing. She suffered in that place. Let her forget it. Be done with it. It's like replaying a horror movie to her. I forbid it!"

"Forbid. . .? To pay back love and kindness? Sometimes even you, Marvin Finell, are wrong! In this case, very wrong. I *am* going to take her to Cedars on Sunday."

"My, my. You *have* become willful. If she has an adverse reaction, you can blame yourself." With those words he switched off the light, turned his back to me, and soon started to snore, without ever giving me his customary goodnight kiss.

Easter Sunday

Stephanie and I attended mass at Blessed Sacrament Catholic Church on Sunset Boulevard. Steven wanted to please Marvin's parents and insisted on being Jewish. He stayed home. The Easter baskets and the boxes of See's candies for the nurses were stowed in the car's trunk.

"Sleeping Beauty! What a pleasant surprise." Dr. Greenberg greeted us with a big smile when we pushed through the glass doors of Cedars. "And how are you?"

He crouched on his heels, the better to lock eyes with Stephanie.

"Hm. . ." Stephanie raised her shoulders, cocking her head to one side while clinging to me. Did she remember him? After she was no longer in the coma, her eyes had always lit up when Dr. Greenberg came into her room.

He held out his arms. She hesitated, then walked a step toward him and answered, "Me. . . fine!"

This was her first partial sentence since her illness.

"How cute you look with your new hairdo, really cute."

"It's easier short," I explained. "She hated having it cut, but with swimming lessons and all—"

"So you're swimming again? What else do you do? Are you taking ballet again?"

Stephanie stuck out her lower lip while pulling down the corners of her mouth, shaking her head.

"We'll begin with that soon," I said. "She needs speech therapy, physical therapy. We don't have a program outlined. Not yet. I wish someone would tell us what would be best for Stephanie."

"She looks marvelous," Dr. Greenberg said as he rose. "Whatever you're doing, it must be the right thing. Keep it up." He gave Stephanie a peck on the cheek and disappeared through double doors.

Whatever you're doing, it must be the right thing.

How often had I heard those words. What we wanted was structure in our lives, a plan for rehabilitation.

Here at Cedars, Stephanie felt her own importance and was filled with compassion as she distributed the Easter baskets to children confined to bed.

Stephanie was allowed in the children's wing, since she had been a patient until recently. Though she was not able to speak, she managed to make herself understood when she communicated in mime with the other children. If Stephanie had bad memories of her hospital stay, they did not surface during this visit. Marvin's fears were unfounded. Perhaps being in a coma proved a blessing in that respect.

Finally I was able to tear Stephanie away from the nurses and children, from being the center of attention, by reminding her that the great Easter egg hunt at the California Yacht Club was waiting—and most important, the rest of the family.

And waiting they were. Impatiently. Marvin, his parents, my mother, Farol, and Steven.

"How did it go?" Marvin asked, the tone of his voice still berating me. Everyone's eyes darted in my direction. I wanted to disappear and grabbed Stephanie's hand a little tighter, afraid she'd become upset. But Stephanie seemed oblivious to our tensions. She flashed a big smile at everyone, breaking the hostile mood.

"Well, Pumpkin, how did you like playing the Easter bunny?" Marvin asked her when she tore herself loose from me and leapt into his arms.

"Hmm, me fine," she said, coquettishly tilting her head and kissing him.

"Dr. Greenberg was there. She loved seeing everyone. Did you notice she spoke a complete sentence?"

We were in bed. Marvin switched off the light and settled into his pillows. Suddenly he asked, "Why did you take her to that place?"

"The hospital?"

"That place, the place where she died."

"Marvin. Stephanie is alive!"

"She died in that goddamned place. My daughter, my Stephanie and all her talents, all she might have become, that Stephanie died there."

I reached for his shoulders and slid closer. "But Marv, the girl she *can* become is very much alive. Alive and asleep in her room." I was desperate to dispense comfort, yet my words had a hollow ring to them. I too had felt this hopelessness. We both grieved the loss of *the* Stephanie, the loss of *the undamaged woman* we would never know.

Marvin buried his face deeper into the pillow, his shoulders shook, the comforter shook, transmitting waves of his pain. A lump in my throat choked me, *What will become of her?* His grief, muffled by pillows, sounded like bellows. He sounded as if he were suffocating. I stroked his hair, massaged his back. "She has improved so much. Didn't you see the sparkle in her eyes today during the egg hunt?" I spoke softly, as if I were speaking to our children when they were hurt. "Remember your mother's comments, 'Stephanie's eyes look so alert, not like the eyes of someone who is brain-damaged.'"

He repeated my last sentence, but finished with, "Not like a *retarded* child."

His words hurt. This was the "R" word I shied away from. I said, "Yes, that's what your mother said. Because she's *not* retarded! Gammy saw it in her eyes. She'll recover and make progress. She'll be all right, I tell you."

"Goddamn your blubbering optimism. I can't talk to you at all."

"It's not good to accept defeat. We have to believe that she'll be all right."

"And believing will make it so? Ha! There is no God up there in heaven who will wave a wand and make it all right. You and your angels and your superstitious beliefs. You can believe all you want; it won't change a damn thing. She's damaged, she's. . ." And again he broke down, sobbing. I hated him at that moment, but I also felt his anguish. I kept stroking his back, but he jerked away.

Chapter Nine

The Teacher

I was told I would not achieve a lot.
I would have to go to special schools.
This woman took me in.
MARIANNE FROSTIG,
a great lady who started a school system
for kids like me. I feel like she's
a part of me; part of my spirit.
She is no longer alive.

—Stephanie Finell, 1987

Summer of 1971

Stephanie needed schooling, and she needed structure in her life. I tried to enroll her in the Fernald School at UCLA but found it would not be an appropriate placement. Many of the children there were more severely handicapped, and in addition, many had serious behavioral problems. I learned there were schools for the blind, schools for the deaf, schools for schizophrenics, and schools for children suffering from cerebral palsy.

There was no school for Stephanie.

Then, I nearly tipped my chair over as I leapt up, pushing the View section of the *Los Angeles Times* across the table, almost knocking over Marvin's orange juice.

"Marv! Look! Read this!" My finger tapped the article, "Here is our hope. Black on white."

"Yes," he agreed after scanning the paper. "This Dr. Frostig might just understand Stephanie's particular problem."

The article described the party, but in its last paragraphs the vocational background of Dr. Marianne Frostig was mentioned. Marianne Frostig began her career in Vienna, in the 1920s, at the College for Social Training where she worked with children at the University of Vienna's Pediatric Clinic. There she encountered hundreds of children who had suffered various degrees of brain damage caused by encephalitis, transmitted by mosquitoes from infected sheep. She was working as a psychiatric social worker, and it appalled Marianne that many of her professors had given up on these children, considering them hopeless cases. Often the parents, embarrassed by having what they considered a *retarded* child in the home, would banish the child to a rear room, out of sight.

Marianne Frostig's attempts to teach these brain-damaged children convinced her that they were capable of learning, *that new pathways in the brain could be made*. Through these children she discovered her own path, and as she later stated: "I therefore decided to devote myself to finding ways to help children with brain damage, even if this exploration were to take a lifetime."

Marvin looked at the rest of the page. "This Dr. Frostig should definitely be consulted," he said, scraping his chair back as he got up to phone the Frostig Center.

I was terribly nervous for our appointment with Dr. Frostig when, several days later, Marvin, Stephanie, and I entered the school near Venice and La Cienega. We pushed through double glass doors into the lobby-reception area. A young teacher accompanied us up the stairs to Dr. Frostig's office.

There sat Dr. Marianne Frostig, looking like the embodiment of a benign Mrs. Claus. Short gray hair, rosy-flushed cheeks, and intense blue eyes—eyes that could not be deceived, eyes that could within a moment's blink change from serious to a twinkle and soften with compassion.

"This is Stephanie? Come here, come," she said, beckoning her with a chubby finger. Steffi went to her, chin to chest. A magnet seemed to draw her close, closer, until she folded within Dr. Frostig's arms, enveloped by the soft creases of a flowery dress and ample flesh.

Stephanie and Marianne Frostig. Neither uttering a sound. Finally Dr. Frostig pointed to a pad of white paper and an assortment of colored pencils. "Do you want to paint me a pretty picture?" she asked.

"Uhuhm. Fine." Stephanie nodded, smiling up at the Mrs. Claus face. She grabbed an orange-colored pencil with her left hand and, holding it awkwardly, drew simple loops.

"Now, tell me all about this child and her illness," Dr. Frostig said, turning to us.

Even though we had told the story so many times, to so many doctors and to many therapists, this time the telling came naturally. I spoke of our problem, explained that we still hadn't found a place where Stephanie could receive remedial training.

"The children in my school have very mild handicaps compared with Stephanie. She does not belong here either," Dr. Frostig said.

I felt as if someone had punched me in the chest. My mouth felt dry and fuzzy, and I could not swallow.

"Now don't look so crestfallen. I said *she doesn't belong* here. I didn't say I wouldn't accept her. Ah, now you smile? Vell. . ." Every so often her lilting Viennese accent became more pronounced. "Vell, I will devise an individual, a special program for Stephanie."

She gave Stephanie a squeeze. Steffi beamed at her.

"I would like for you to bring her here every day, for half an hour. I will work with her personally. I will observe her, design a therapeutic plan for her, and once she is able, she may come for longer hours. Hopefully, she'll be able to attend regular classes soon. All right, Stephanie?"

"Right. Fine," Stephanie answered. *Right.* A new word.

When, minutes later we walked out through the lobby, I felt weightless as if I were one of the sunbeams streaming through the windows. The floor, the carpet, all had disappeared beneath my feet. If I could have painted us the way I felt at that moment, I would have painted us hovering ten feet above the ground, floating through the glass doors into a world bathed in a golden light, while my heart sang, *We found someone who cares, we found someone who cares!*

But more important, we found someone eminently qualified to help Stephanie.

We later learned more of Marianne Frostig's past. She married a neuropsychiatrist in Vienna and devised new methods to help him run a psychiatric hospital in Poland. The Frostigs' success with patients became widely known. They used methods to transform inactive patients in custodial care to become integrated in work and independent living. In 1938 their reputation brought them an offer from a California mental hospital in Camarillo, near Los Angeles. Their move to the United States proved their salvation, as the following year Germany invaded Poland. After the Nazis' occupation from September 1939 onward, everyone at the hospital the Frostigs had worked in, individual patients as well as staff, were killed.

Marianne's husband worked at the hospital in Camarillo but was not granted a medical license for private practice until 1947. In order to further her career, Marianne returned to academe, earning a doctorate in psychology at USC, also in 1947. After her husband's death in 1958, Marianne became the breadwinner for the family, which had grown to include a son and a daughter.

Marianne opened a school out of a house she bought on Fairfax Boulevard. From those humble beginnings she moved on to operate a school on Melrose Boulevard. She had now begun applying her own methods, and by the time the Frostig Center moved to the school on Venice Boulevard where we met her, Marianne Frostig had become a recognized authority on teaching children with dyslexia, which was often accompanied by physical coordination problems. Her goal was to enable these children eventually to return to regular classrooms. The Frostig method became known globally. Governments sent teachers from as far away as Sri Lanka and Chile to learn Dr. Frostig's techniques. The current Marianne Frostig Center is located in Pasadena, California.

And Marianne Frostig was willing to help our daughter.

In the parking lot Marvin said, "Let's celebrate, Snorg." He called Stephanie by one of the many silly names he often made up. "Where do you want to eat?"

Stephanie pulled up her shoulders, cocked her head, and smiled.

"Okay, that's fine with me," he answered her shrug. "That's where we'll go. The Bantam Cock it is."

We knew all the waiters. They had commiserated with us during Stephanie's hospital stay when Marvin and I lunched there almost daily. We walked over to Benny's station. His smile, flashes of white in his black face, stretched across his cheeks.

"My, do we e'er look pretty, little Miss Stephanie!" Benny hugged her. She turned her cheek for a kiss and then kissed him back, a big loud smack.

When we left the restaurant, I still felt a warm glow. "Marv? I would like to thank Someone. You know? I would very much like to stop by the church. . .the one on Sunset—light a candle—it's not far. You mind?"

"No, I don't mind. I'll read the paper. You go and do your thing."

Stephanie and I entered the semi-dark church. The nave was almost empty. We knelt in front of the Christ mosaic and lit a seven-day candle. The flame flickered and appeared as tiny golden points in Stephanie's brown eyes. I ran my hand over my child's hair, drew her a little closer. My entire being felt wide-open—almost painfully so—with love and gratitude.

"Dr. Fostik, Dr. Fostik!" Stephanie skipped, ran, and almost tripped when she saw the friendly shape appear in the hallway. She collided with her, hugged her, and followed Marianne Frostig into one of the small rooms used in a one-on-one situation. When Stephanie closed the door behind herself, she did not look back.

I was not in the room with them for Stephanie's half-hour of retraining of the brain and therefore did not know what the lessons entailed, but I could tell by

Stephanie's happiness each time she saw Dr. Frostig that loving the teacher was the most important element in her ability to learn.

By the middle of July, Stephanie had learned a few sentences. She relearned her native tongue as others might learn a foreign language. At first she used nouns and pronouns, then verbs—mostly in the imperative—leaving out adverbs, prepositions, and conjunctions, the connecting links creating fluidity of language.

"Celia, put me car," she would say.

I corrected her, "*Celia, please put me in the car.*"

"Celia, please put me car."

"No. Stephanie, repeat: Celia, please put me *in the* car. *In the car.*"

"In the car, in the car."

"Okay, Stephanie, now the whole sentence. *Celia, please put me in the car.* Repeat it."

"Celia, please. . .put me. . .in the car." She giggled.

"Yes. Good. Now again—"

And on it went.

This effort of rerouting her brain-paths cost Stephanie an enormous amount of energy. At night she would sink into bed exhausted and drift off to sleep within seconds.

When the fall term began, she went to school for two full hours every day.

Eventually the Frostig Center cured Stephanie of her drooling. She sniffed ammonia, which she hated—sucked on lemons, which she liked—sucked up confetti-type paper bits with a straw and deposited these, using mouth-muscle control, as patterns onto white paper. All these exercises and therapies helped redevelop the partially paralyzed, insensate interior of Stephanie's mouth. And gradually, Stephanie stopped drooling, began writing, and doing simple arithmetic again.

One of the Frostig methods concerning arithmetic particularly impressed me. Many children with learning disabilities had over time, while competing in regular classrooms, developed inferiority complexes. Many came from broken homes or from dysfunctional families. Others came from homes of poverty. These children did not want anything *taken away* from them. Dr. Frostig's method made a game out of subtraction. Rather than take two from five—two eggs hatched and changed into two chicks. If there were five eggs, how many eggs now? How many chicks?

And along with the other children, Stephanie flourished.

Stephanie and I went back to Rancho Los Amigos for additional evaluations and for a follow-up EEG. This revealed a slight spiking of certain electrical impulses in her brain. She had to remain on the anti-convulsing medication, Dilantin.

I worried about the medication. So far Stephanie was free of any adverse symptoms, but we had been warned it might cause excessive hair growth on arms and legs. Worse, it would in time cause inflamed and bleeding gums and lead eventually to periodontal problems, with probable loss of teeth. But at this point the doctors were reluctant to change Dilantin for a milder medication.

Stephanie's speech had progressed; and she brought strange and scraggly drawings home from school, which she proudly showed us.

When alone in our bedroom, I paused in front of the self-portrait she had made when she was only six years old, in second grade, before her illness. This large crayon collage on white paper showed her wearing a dress made from calico, holding our two West Highland terriers on a leash. She drew her favorite red boots, laced up in a late nineteenth-century style—all drawn in great detail. Comparing this to her present artwork, I could not help but feel saddened. *She will improve, she will improve*, I told myself.

It was time for our first parents' meeting with Marianne Frostig. "Ah, the Finells!" She greeted us with outstretched arms and led us into her office.

She pulled a large piece of paper from her desk drawer. This squiggly mass of crayon lines showed a large rabbit carrying a smaller one in its stomach, and a still smaller rabbit within it, and a still smaller rabbit within that one. Four rabbits in all.

"Stephanie drew these. . .and. . ." She searched in her drawer and pulled out another piece of paper. "I've kept the first one she drew." She held up the simple squiggle drawing. "And now," she pointed to the rabbits. "This! Is it not wonderful?"

Pregnant rabbits. Marvin took the drawing from my hand and examined it. "Does she know something I don't know?" he asked, looking at me.

Dr. Frostig's blue eyes also twinkled at the question.

"No, no, I'm not pregnant." I felt myself blush. "Maybe it's Steff's wishful thinking. Wanting a little sister." After Stephanie's birth, I had wanted to have more children but did not get pregnant. At this time I did not want another child. Maybe in another year, but at this point I would feel as if I were betraying Stephanie. She needed my undivided attention.

It was time for us to leave. "Don't let her get lazy," Dr. Frostig said as she shook my hand goodbye. "Have her use her right hand daily. She's made great progress. Vell? We'll see you again soon. . ."

The words of Henry Adams came to mind, *A teacher affects eternity: he can never tell where his influence stops*. Marianne Frostig was a teacher who had a profound effect on others' lives. Stephanie loved her and would never forget her. We had found our salvation in her teaching.

Chapter Ten

Patterns and Repetition

Loneliness begins when I'm alone in my bedroom
I feel like a spot on the wall.

—Stephanie Finell

It was the summer of '72, and Stephanie had made excellent progress. Her speech was almost back to that of a normal eight-year-old. During Steven's stay in summer camp, Marvin took Stephanie and me on a business trip to Hawaii. We stayed at the Kahala Hilton, in a suite on the top floor, overlooking the man-made lagoon where dolphins performed.

"What pretty fish, Mom," Stephanie said when she saw the dolphins leap through hoops.

"Lesson number one: Stephanie, dolphins are not fish. They're mammals, warm blooded."

"But Mom. . .they live in water."

I proceeded to tell her how evolution took separate species on different paths.

She was not convinced. "Mom. . .if they breathe like a dog or like people, then how come they swim underwater?"

"Well, Steffi, you hold your breath for a long time when you swim the sixty feet of our pool underwater. A dolphin has adapted to his environment, and he can hold his breath for much, much longer."

I wrapped my arm around her small shoulders as we stood on the balcony, watching the dolphins breaking to the surface and crowning themselves with leis of frangipani.

We'd arrived in Honolulu at midday. Now Marvin waited impatiently for us to change. He was free to spend the rest of the day with us. After seeing the dolphins, Stephanie couldn't wait to put on her bathing suit and inspect the animals up close, on our way to the beach.

A narrow bridge spanned one end of the dolphin pool. "Steffi, not so fast, you'll fall!" I shouted as she ran on ahead. Her terry robe flapped. She was about to lose her right sandal, and she tripped but caught herself and continued to run, now crossing the bridge, while looking over her shoulder to where the dolphins swam, and—oops! She fell, splash, into the dolphin pool.

One of the dolphins swam to her side in a flash, nudging her, pushing her gently. She held out her hand, the dolphin mouthed her fingers. I feared the robe would become water-soaked and drag her down and made ready to jump to the rescue, when I felt Marvin's hand on my arm.

"She's safe. She swims like a fish herself. Don't worry. Look, she's so happy. Give her another minute."

Stephanie whirled as two dolphins swam circles around her. Fun or not, swimming in the dolphin pool was strictly against the rules, and I worried we'd get into trouble. "Stephanie, come out of there. You might scare the dolphins. Come back here," I coaxed. She shook her head.

"Please Mommy, I love it, I love it."

"You can't stay in there. One of the trainers will come and get angry."

"Okay, Mom," she finally agreed. Then, taking a loud deep breath, she dove. The water was murky, and for a moment I couldn't see her as she swam beneath a dolphin. The dolphin appeared to smile when he—or she—turned, looked me straight in the eye, and—also dove. And then, Stephanie, plus dolphin, surfaced together. Laughing.

The lawyer in Marvin Finell got the better of him and he commanded, "Snorg, come here right now!" Stephanie turned, swam to the edge without effort, despite the weight of her soaked robe. Marv leaned over and helped her climb out.

"Wow, that was such fun, Mom. Oh boy, just great."

"Come. . ." I tugged at her arm, as she kept turning, not willing to take her eyes off the animals.

"Mom, my flip-flop. . ." she cried out, pointing to one of them floating on the surface.

"I'll get it," Marvin said, kneeling on the bridge. He stretched his arm to reach the sandal and. . .he fell into the pool. The dolphins did not swim to him, they kept their distance, watching. He quickly climbed out, wet and apologetic. We were still laughing at the dolphin adventure, when our lunch was served near the beach.

Quickly the summer of 1972 slipped away. More than a year and a half had passed since Stephanie's illness. She had made much progress, but still, her brain damage shadowed our daily family life.

All this was interspersed with idyllic moments. Steven spent several weeks at Catalina Island Boys' Camp, where we visited him while our sailboat, an

Ericson sloop we had named *Ariel* (after the spirit of the air in Shakespeare's play *The Tempest*) lay moored in Cat Harbor.

For a few weeks we seemed to live in a Norman Rockwell picture: Stephanie holding her fishing rod at the stern; Steven paddling about in the dinghy, and I, sitting on the hatch playing my guitar. Suddenly Stephanie pulled up her rod, and lo and behold, seven silvery fish were dangling from salami-baited hooks. She counted them and shouted again and again, "I caught seven fish, seven little fish." Her face was radiant as she watched them wiggle. It surprised me that she didn't get upset when we told her they had to be released, all seven were too small.

A few weeks later and before the children would have to return to school, Marvin took us along on a business trip to Seattle. Our suite was on the thirty-ninth floor—the "London Suite," in the Washington Plaza Hotel. Puget Sound lay in the distance like a polished tray of silver. Dark forests leaned against purple mountains, defining the lavender of sky.

Stephanie and I sat by the picture window and watched the sun turning the water to bronze. Stephanie said, "Look Mom, they look like toy boats in a bathtub," pointing to the ferryboats, tiny shapes in the distance, crisscrossing the Sound.

Early the next morning an eiderdown blanket of fog covered all, creating illusions. A lone ferryboat appeared to be climbing the sky enveloped in fog.

We visited Blake Island on Labor Day. Tourist time: Indian hut, Indian meal, Indian dances, baked salmon and mountain-blackberry pie. The lunch had been eaten, the dances watched, and I sat on a tree stump on the grass. Both Steven and Stephanie were louder than usual. Where was Marvin? How far had he walked? Suddenly, the bushes broke behind me.

"Rroah booh!" He growled, grabbing me.

I jumped. "Don't do that to me! I thought you were a bear or a moose!"

"Don't be silly!" He swirled me around, grinning like a mischievous boy. "Just us lions roaming the woods," he laughed, referring to his zodiac sign, Leo. And he added, "Have they calmed down? Where are they?"

"There!" I pointed to the children playing at the water's edge. "They've been quiet now for exactly one minute. Well. . .perhaps two. Fight, fight, fight, about every little thing. Who gets which stone, which pebble, which piece of driftwood. They're driving me insane."

"Steven. . .that's. . ., well. . ., but I'm surprised Steff's becoming so aggressive. Maybe she feels the need to assert herself."

"Perhaps it's a good sign." I shrugged. "But it does not make for a tranquil summer's day." I paused, then said, "Marv, I'd like to be alone for a few minutes. Recharge my batteries. Mind watching the kids? I won't be long."

He nodded. "There's a nice place down the path, right after that big log."

I followed his directions and found a small meadow, an oasis of peace beneath towering trees. I lay down in the grass and buried my face in its freshness, inhaling the plain dank goodness of earth. I closed my eyes and tuned in to the sounds of nature. The cawing of crows, the flute song of a bird, the strummed melody of a grasshopper. When I opened my eyes, I noticed a gossamer spider's web in a branch, inches from me, catching the gold of day in a dew drop, refracting it in a myriad of sparkles before the dark tableau of trees, while sunlight slipped off leaves, coating them in ever so many shades of green.

Later we all took a walk by the water, where logs, bleached gray like ancient whalebones, had washed up on the sand. The children no longer fought. They climbed, laughed, shrieked while Marvin and I sat and watched the sun's rippling reflections on the stained-glass sea.

That evening we ordered room service while sitting by the windows watching the sun burn the sky. At the edge, the water still glowed like red-hot steel smelting in a furnace, a minute later it had turned to burnished copper, and then dissolved into the gray of slate. Abruptly, the mountains swallowed the sun. The show was over.

In the morning, the thick fog of Puget Sound was punctured by the deep bellows of foghorns and the tinkling of ship's bells. Television had proclaimed Labor Day to be America's last fling at summer. Seattle proved television to be right.

With the gray day and the drizzle came the shocking news of the murder of Israeli athletes by Palestinian terrorists at the Olympic Games in Munich. What we watched on television, made me shout, "Oh no! Not again! Again Jews are being killed in Germany."

Martin put his hand on my quivering shoulders and said, "This time though they are Palestinians doing the killing. And the Germans are stopping it as best they can. Don't cry. . ." He spoke gently when he saw how emotional I was.

I wiped my eyes and my nose. "This is such a crazy world. There are so many mad, mad people in it."

Prompted by the events on television, I tried to explain to our children what Adolf Hitler and the Nazis had done to human beings during his Third Reich. I did not know much of child psychology at the time, and how inappropriate it was for them to hear the facts of history at their age, it would only frighten them. "Ha! The Reich that was supposed to last a mythical Thousand Years. Can you imagine the whole world taken over by the Nazis? Fortunately it lasted only twelve years." I then told them that Hitler had systematically killed Jews and gypsies, and others who were infirm and born with handicaps.

Stephanie asked, "How come they didn't kill you, Mommy?"

"I'm not Jewish, Stephanie."

"Would they have killed me? I'm Jewish."

"Me? Would they have killed me?" Steven asked.

"Steven, this is difficult to explain, but they would have killed all of us if I had been married to your father then, and we'd have been a family in Germany. Then they would have killed me too."

"Why? You said they wouldn't have killed you because you're not Jewish."

"But Steven, had I been married, I would have stuck by my family. In many cases they sent everyone in a family to a concentration camp."

"Hold it Karin. Just hold it—" Marvin cut in, making a gesture for me to be quiet. "I don't think they would have killed the children."

"Marvin! The children have to know the truth. You joined the Army at age seventeen to fight the Nazis. You knew the evil that went on." I felt sick with guilt for being German and the vagaries of what might have been had we all been born at a different time in a different place. Marvin placed his hand on my mouth now, seeing the frightened look in his children's eyes. Finally I understood, *Yes, they are too young to be told the truth.*

The weather outside our windows made everything beyond the glass appear shrouded in a dismal gloom. It echoed the gray hopelessness I felt for the murder and violence rampant on this globe.

Again we sat by the window. Puget Sound was now a dull cookie sheet with ferryboats crisscrossing like flies searching for sugar. My earlier mood of oneness with all had shattered into fragments—like the rose-colored vase we had bought on our honeymoon in Venice, which slipped from my hands just before this trip.

We were back in our house on Ridgedale Drive. Steven and I were having lunch. He had spent the night with his friend Tom Hand (son of Anne, our connection to Marianne Frostig) who was home for Christmas from a boarding school in Arizona.

When we finished eating, Steven got up and carried the dishes to the sink. Then he turned, holding on to the back of the Windsor chair. He stuck his jutting chin out a little farther, which made him look like a boy version of Orson Wells.

"Mom? I want to go to Treehaven with Tom."

"You want to. . .what? Boarding school? Steven, you're much too young."

"I'll be ten in a month. Please, Mom, I want to get away. I hate my school."

"El Rodeo is one of the best schools. . .It's the main reason we moved to this address."

"I want to go away. Tom said—"

"Steven, your friends are here. You don't know anyone in Tucson. Only Tom."

He fidgeted, walked to the refrigerator, and pulled a Coke from the shelf. "The teachers here don't like me. The kids are all stuck up. I want to get away. . .

for a while. . ." His voice became almost inaudible. "And I don't like being around Stephanie all the time. I don't like having a retarded sister."

I looked at him in shock. *A retarded sister.* He'd called Stephanie a mental retard before, but he was not name-calling her now.

"Steve, haven't you noticed the progress she's made, how much the Frostig Center has helped her?" His face remained set in that bulldog look. "Steven, she isn't retarded. In some ways she's very intelligent. Her speech is improving, almost back to normal." I couldn't continue. I left the kitchen for a supply of tissues.

"But, Mom," he said when I returned. "Stephanie can't even find the bathroom anywhere. Every place we go she has to be helped." His voice rose, got shrill. "She's very retarded!"

"I don't understand you. This from the boy who tried to nurse a wounded bird back to life? Who always worries about the dogs? Can't you have the same compassion for your own sister? She needs all of us to help her back to a normal life."

I cursed my tears, while damp tissues dotted the floor. I tried to convince him. "Steve, you know she's a lot better. So what if we still help her find a bathroom in a restaurant, big deal! What if she were in a wheelchair, and you'd have to help push it? What then? We have to be so very grateful she's progressed as far as—" I had to swallow hard.

I mentioned it to Marvin after dinner. "Independent little shit. Hey, he's your son, lady!"

"He's as much yours as he's mine." My voice turned to ice. "I've been thinking about it all afternoon. Steven has been taking a back seat in our family lately. Maybe we should look into it. Can we afford it?"

"That's not the point. I think he'd get a better education right here in our school district. Right here, living with us."

"Perhaps the desert air would be good for him. He's had these asthma attacks again. Oh, didn't I tell you? Dr. Rosin put him on medication. You didn't—"

"When did he see Dr. Rosin?"

"Yesterday. You came home so late I forgot to tell you. He had an Adrenalin shot."

"My guess it's psychosomatic."

"Whatever the reason, a different environment might be good for him. He wouldn't need his psychologist any longer. That would pay for some of the tuition right there."

"I told you it's not the money I'm worried about."

"We could call Tom's parents and find out about Treehaven from them. Contact the school and check things out. No? We could be open to it. Perhaps it would be a solution."

"Let's go to bed. I'll sleep on it."

I felt torn. I knew I would miss Steven. I would like for him to live with us so that we could have a daily influence on his upbringing. But I also wanted him to be happy.

Late January 1973

The desert air—crisp, bracing, cool, like astringent aftershave lotion—hit our faces as the doors to the plane opened and we descended the aluminum landing stairs. Steven skipped ahead of us, skipped across the black tarmac into what he believed would be his very own adventure.

A week earlier, the four of us, including Stephanie, had traveled to Tucson, inspected the school, and met with the principal and the teachers. Steven found Treehaven as Tom had described it. He entered the school two weeks before his tenth birthday.

When his letters arrived, they were full of enthusiasm. *I have a chicken,* he wrote. *A Rhode Island rooster named Henry. And there are pigs here down the road. They are big and pink like you-can-eat-'em pigs.*

I chuckled when I read this to Stephanie. We both remembered what he had written from Catalina Island Boy's Camp the year before. *There are boars here. Boars are like pigs, only piggier.*

Steven went horseback riding on mountain trails. I hoped that by being close to nature, his own volcanic nature would be moderated.

Spring turned into summer. Stephanie went to summer school. Steven came home on vacation. Then Steven invited Hendryk, who lived in a Hollywood canyon, to go fishing with him to the Santa Monica pier. I drove them down the almost ten miles and dropped them off with their fishing gear. Steven had a few dollars on him for the two to take the bus home and buy refreshments and worms for bait while at the pier.

Several hours later the doorbell rang. An exhausted and sweaty Hendryk stood at the door. Steven had abandoned him soon after they reached the pier and refused to give him any money or coins either to call me or his mother or take a bus back to Los Angeles. The poor kid had walked the ten miles or so in the summer's heat. And where was Steven?

I drove Hendryk home. His mother worked in a school teaching German nearby. I called her and then took Hendryk to her school. It had been Steven's invitation to go fishing. I was hardly back in the house when my mother called. Steven had walked from the pier to her house. I was livid, abandoning his friend without a penny so far from home. What kind of a friend was Steven?

Then my mother told me. Steven had a big fight with Hendryk, who taunted him for being clumsy in baiting the hooks. Hendryk called him a mental retard, "Just like your sister." That's what he said. That did it. Steven hit him, pushed him down, and left with the fishing rods and the money.

Mother, who lived close to the beach, asked if she should bring Steven home. I was angry. Even if Hendryk had called him names, it still was a dastardly thing to do to a friend. Now it would seem, former friend.

"If you have time I'd appreciate it if you'd bring him; I don't even want to look him in the eye at this time."

"Don't be so harsh with him, Karin. He's just a little boy and it is very difficult for him to handle this situation. He always takes the back seat to his sister."

"I can't forgive Steven's disloyal behavior toward his friend. That's inexcusable."

Then there were the renewed worries about Stephanie. She was vomiting a great deal of late, often when in the car, going to or coming from school. I believed that some of her nausea was related to nervous tension. She was becoming increasingly aware of herself and of her limitations.

Stephanie was happiest in her new ballet class in Santa Monica. But here too she remained in the beginners' group for session after session.

"Lift, point, close. Lift, point, close. Lift to the side. . .Stephanie, *attencion*—" The mistress of the ballet school, Mahri glided on small feet across the parquet floor and tapped her on the rear, using a slender willow stick. "And lift to the side." Stephanie jerked her body straight, maneuvered her feet, and Mahri, who had been reprimanding her a moment ago, smiled and said, "Very good, that's it, Stephanie, and. . .close to the back."

Occasionally, Cloris Leachman participated in the lessons, clad like the others in leotards, having joined her eight-year-old daughter's class to get some exercise herself. After the lesson, Cloris came over to me and, pointing to Stephanie, said, "It's amazing. I've known your daughter only for a short while, but I can really see progress. She's doing great."

Those moments were my rewards. I myself often did not notice the minuscule advances Stephanie made. If a stranger noticed an improvement and told me about it, it lightened my load.

At Mahri's school Stephanie met Hugi—"Little Sister," as her Hungarian family called her. She was a vivacious, giggly girl with impish eyes and dark brown bangs cut straight across her forehead. Soon the two became friends, and Hugi spent a great deal of time at our house.

Hugi entered Stephanie's life at the same time as Michelle did from the Frostig Center. Little by little her former El Rodeo schoolmates showed other interests and stopped seeing her—much as the *not-tcherman* doctor had predicted.

It was the night before Stephanie's tenth birthday. Marvin came into my study, carrying scissors, saying, "Please? Cut some flowers to take to Steff in the morning."

"Something's wrong with my typewriter." I said, pounding my fist on the desk in frustration. Since I had given up my studies at UCLA (two courses and a thesis short of my PhD), I wrote articles and worked on a screenplay. An article for a German literary geographic magazine, *MERIAN*, was due in a week. "It's stuck or something," I explained. "Can't you please cut the flowers?"

Marvin returned holding a screwdriver in his hand and busied himself. *Okay, he wants me to cut the flowers.* I went out in the dark, gathered a bouquet of yellow chrysanthemums, and as I was carrying them in a glass, my allergies acted up and I sneezed all the way up the stairs.

We had bought a charm for her, and now I placed this little fish of gold resting in a silver box among the star-faced flowers. I visualized Stephanie's smile the next morning, when we'd surprise her, singing, "Happy Birthday, to you," carrying blossoms and presents. Again, I was keenly aware of how fortunate we were to be able to light ten candles on our daughter's birthday cake.

God's Tears
fall from heaven
down-to-earth
tears from God's eyes
HE is sad when so many children die

When one child dies
for no apparent reason
a shoot-out
or starvation
or when evil people kill a child
That's when God cries

Young and old,
trust in your heart
and not in your head.

Protect your children
love your children
for God is all things

HE or SHE knows
that loving ALL is the answer

The children of the world
are neither good nor bad
love is the GOOD

—Stephanie Finell

Chapter Eleven

The Goldfish Bowl

Protect your children/ Love your children. . .
—Stephanie Finell

March 1974

Stephanie's progress had been steady, though it was slower than I hoped. Her speech was that of a normal ten-year-old. Again, she was popular with her classmates—now from the Frostig Center—and was invited to many birthday parties, prompting frequent visits to the toy store.

I was in a hurry. I'd been in the toy store only for a few minutes to pick up presents I had already bought and I left Stephanie in the car. Where is my car? Where did the attendant park it? Ah, there. I spotted the car partially hidden behind a van at the far end of the lot.

At that moment the parking attendant closed the door to the driver's side and slinked off. I ran, not knowing why. He also ran. In the opposite direction.

I opened the car door and saw Stephanie's zipper was open, her jeans and panties pulled below her hips; and her leather belt had been thrown onto the back seat. She clutched a dollar bill in her left hand. I stared, confused as to what was going on.

"Stephanie! What. , .why are your pants down?"

"Mommy!" Sobs drowned her voice, making it difficult for me to understand the words she blurted out. "The man called me a boy!"

"The man who parked the car?"

"He said he'd give me a dollar if I was a girl!"

She trembled as tears rolled down her cheeks. Her hands pushed furiously at her recently acquired super-short bob. "I hate my hair, I hate it. See!" She pointed her finger at me. "The man thought I'm a boy!"

I screamed at attendant. "Hey, you!" The man turned and looked at me, an alarmed smirk smeared across his face. His thin mustache quivered, his mouth twitched. "You!" I repeated, "Yes, I mean you. Come over here!"

He skulked toward me. His wire-rimmed glasses slid down his nose, he held his head slightly forward and cocked to the left, his right arm raised to shoulder height, ready to fend off an imaginary blow. "Yes? Ma'am?" he lisped, his voice a thin falsetto.

"Is this the man, Stephanie?"

"Yes, Mommy." Stephanie took one quick look, then hid her head in the crook of her arm.

"What did you do to my daughter?"

"Me? No do noathing. Honor, me no do none." He stood like a trapped animal.

"I asked you, What did you do? What kind of a pervert are you?" Now why did I say that? I wanted to choke him. Instead I pushed the dollar into his face. "And this?"

"Honest! Me 'ave wife, me children. You believe. *He* must 'a' found the dollar in street. *Si*, in street. *He* must 'a' found—I no do—"

I threw the dollar at the attendant, slid behind the wheel, turned the ignition, and gunned the motor. As I shot past him, brushing his clothes, I thought, *Stupid man, calling Stephanie "he."* In the rearview mirror, I saw him give me the finger.

My tires squealed onto Camden Drive, I crossed Santa Monica Boulevard on orange turning red, then came to a screeching halt at the stop sign at Elevado, nearly hitting a teenager on a bicycle. The sudden stop made Stephanie bang her head on the windshield. In my rage I'd forgotten to put on her seat belt. Her pants were still down. I took a deep breath. Stephanie had curled into a small knot. She huddled against the door, pressing her head against the window. Tears were rolling down her cheeks. I reached over to pull up her pants, buckled her in, hugged her, kissed her. "Sweetheart, don't cry. I didn't hit the kid."

"No. But Mommy, the man's a liar. He said I found the dollar in the street. I wasn't even in the street."

"Honey, I believe you. Don't cry. Please. Things will be all right. I'll drive nice and slow, and when we get home, we'll have a little cake and milk. A Kaffeeklatch. We'll forget that horrible man."

Her voice was a whisper. "Okay, Mommy."

I dialed Marvin's office. "Marv? No, no. No one is hurt—" Then I told him what had happened.

A young police officer arrived to take the report. He got there before Marvin. I found out I'd made a mistake in throwing the dollar at the man, every little bit counts as evidence. The officer kept referring to Stephanie as *the victim*. The word made me shudder. He also told us to see a doctor immediately.

"But officer, he did not come near her sexually, if that is what the examination would determine."

"In these cases, the victim has to be seen by a doctor at once."

We sat in the waiting room of a physician who specialized in rape and molestation cases. Stephanie crouched low, mesmerized by goldfish swimming in circles in an oversized round glass bowl on the coffee table.

I looked at Stephanie and froze. It was as if my child's sweet face was caught in the fishbowl. Trapped. Her face appeared in the water, and small orange fish swam over her eyes, her flattened nose, her slightly opened mouth. Her features were stretched out of proportion by the glass, like the optical illusions in mirrored rooms at a carnival. The small hairs on my arms stood straight up.

The door opened, and Dr. Thornton ushered us into her office. She seemed to be a compassionate woman in her early fifties with graying hair, sensible shoes, and a broad smile. She radiated sympathy. After I briefly informed her of Stephanie's medical history and the incident in the parking lot, she asked me to wait outside while she examined Stephanie.

Marvin stormed through the door just as I'd returned to my seat in the waiting room. I could feel his anger as a radiating force. After a short while, Stephanie stepped through the door. Dr. Thornton took note of Marvin, his sparse hair flying upward, and she noticed my wet eyes.

"Now, now. Calm yourselves. Both of you. Please, there is no reason. Everything is fine. Right, Steffi?" She gave her a hug and directed her toward the couch. "You have a lovely young lady here. Stephanie is all right. If you two would come in with me?"

"The hymen is intact," the doctor said, closing the door behind us.

"It should be. He didn't have time for—"

"There are scratches around the vagina. These could be self-inflicted. However, I think it was very lucky that you were not very long in that shop. The scratches might have been inflicted by the molester." The doctor paused. "He might have been able to break her hymen."

"What?" I cried out, not quite understanding what I heard.

"But he didn't," she went on. "I don't think Stephanie suffered psychological trauma. She views the world very simply. There was no pleasure, there was no fear, only a certain revulsion at the man and anger about being thought of as a boy. I don't think Stephanie will have any guilt connected with this experience. You are lucky in having an emotionally well-adjusted daughter." She paused, looked at her notes. "She's a miracle, really, from what I see here concerning her bout with encephalitis. Amazing child."

"If this case goes to court, do you think we stand a chance to have this sicko locked up?" Marvin asked.

"Molestation cases are very difficult to prosecute. After examining her, I could testify that she is unable to zip her pants up or down and unable to take the belt off by herself. That's all I could testify to. You're a lawyer, Mr. Finell. I need not remind you that the burden to prove the man's guilt lies with the prosecution."

"I want that man in jail." Marvin got up and prowled the floor. He stopped, grabbed the back of a chair so hard his knuckles showed white. "I'm worried about the psychological effect this whole thing might have on Stephanie."

I squirmed, nodded.

"The procedures leading up to the trial will most likely produce some temporary behavioral changes," Dr. Thornton said. "Stephanie has led a protected life. Suddenly she becomes the center of attention. With the police, the DA, maybe even in her school. The two of you will measure every word said in front of her and what effect it might have. The atmosphere between you will become charged. Tense. Of course it will affect Stephanie."

Marvin and I looked at each other, aware that fate again had placed us on a tightrope.

We returned home. A few minutes later Detective Marilyn Graber arrived. She was a woman in her early thirties, with shoulder-length chestnut hair, dressed in a navy business suit and medium heels. I liked her immediately. She tried to put us at ease, walked toward the built-in bookcases, reading the books' titles on the spines.

"Ah, I see poetry, drama, history, psychology, and politics. His and hers, huh?" She smiled as she walked to the sofa and let herself sink into the soft cushions.

Marvin said, "Karin was an English major and I—"

"You're interested in everything," I cut in.

"I was an English major myself," Detective Graber said. "Before Police Academy. UCLA."

"Really? That's my old Alma Mater." I smiled at the coincidence.

The room opened to the entry hall. Steven, home for a holiday, rushed past and up the stairs like a veritable hurricane, caught himself in mid-ascent, peered into the living room, and slid down the stairs on the seat of his pants.

"Hi Steve!" I motioned in his direction. "Marilyn, this is our son, Steven."

"Yeah, hi! Celia said there's a detective here. Where is he?"

"That's me. Glad to meet you. I'm Detective Graber with the Beverly Hills Police." She held out her hand.

Steven took her hand and shook it in an exaggerated fashion. "I'm Steve Finell, with the Los Angeles Police. Lieutenant Finell!"

"Steve, don't be a wise guy. You owe Detective Graber an apology," Marvin said.

"Really? You're *really* a cop? A girl?" He swirled the word *girl* around the back of his throat, as if it were an unpronounceable word. "I thought that was only on *Mod Squad.*"

"Nope, young man. In fact there are some crime investigations in which a woman can make more headway than a man. Want to see my credentials?" Marilyn Graber opened her purse. Stephanie, freshly bathed and dressed in robe and slippers sauntered into the room and sidled up to the detective. The children stared wide-eyed at Marilyn Graber as she pulled a pair of handcuffs and a small gun out of her bag.

Both children reacted with a loud, "Wow!"

Steven's face now reflected a measure of respect. "Do you ever use that stuff, I mean the handcuffs and all that?"

"Yes, I'm sorry to say, ever so often."

"Do you. . .sometimes shoot people?" Stephanie asked.

"Shut up," Steven shouted, shoving her. "What're you doing here anyway? It's past your bedtime! Up, Stephanie!"

"You don't have to boss me around!" Stephanie yelled back, stomping the hardwood floor.

"As a matter of fact, Detective Graber is here because of Stephanie," I told Steven. "Maybe you can leave us alone for a bit. I'll explain later."

"Are you gonna put handcuffs on Steff and lock her up?" Steven grinned.

"Steve, you heard your mother. Go to your room, we'll talk later."

Steven left, his head bent low to his chest. I felt sorry for my little boy. His sister had taken center stage again. I left my chair and went to him, putting my arm around his shoulders.

"Stevie," I whispered, "something has happened to Stephanie. A bad man tried to do bad things to her. I'll tell you later, okay?" I gave him a little kiss on the cheek, which he wiped off with the back of his hand, as he shook himself free and raced up the stairs.

Marvin explained Stephanie's medical history to Marilyn Graber and the reason why she could not have unzipped her pants.

The detective turned to Stephanie, "Honey, may I ask you a few questions?"
"Okay!"
"Did the man ask you where you live?"
"Yep. I told him."
I sucked in my breath.
"I told him, none of your bees wax!"
I exhaled a loud breath of relief.

Later, we kissed the children good night. I told each their own favorite story, stories I had made up for them. Now I felt worn-out, tired, and I needed some quiet time. I lit a fire in the fireplace, fell onto the bed, and listened to the soft cadences of Mozart's twenty-first Piano Concerto. Marvin returned with a tray of steaming mugs of cappuccino. He placed the tray on the bed, kissed me gently on the neck. "I don't know if we should talk about it now," Marvin said, reluctant to break the mellow mood. "But I've been thinking. . .I think we ought to press for prosecution."

"What if it's damaging to her?"

"Steffi is strong. I think she can handle it."

I wondered where Marvin rushed to so early the next morning. He wasn't dressed for the office, not wearing khaki pants and a polo shirt. When he came back an hour later, his shirt showed small sprinkles of red drops. His face wore a sheepish expression.

He admitted he hadn't listened to anyone and had acted like a fool. He'd parked his car on Camden Drive. There he stood and watched from inside a phone booth, located between the "76" gas station and the toy store's parking lot. And he waited. He said that the description Stephanie and I had given Detective Graber ran through his mind like a film—a slightly out of focus film. He jumped when he saw the first attendant arrive. Latino, short, plump. No, he remembered that I had described the man as scrawny, wearing glasses.

Then he arrived. Marvin's breath now came in short gasps, as if he were reliving the incident while he was telling it. "My body felt as if it were a car and some force pressed down hard on the gas pedal. As if my body were accelerating and wanted to jump out of itself."

He related how *the man* crossed toward the ticket booth, opened the door, and, standing by the entrance, pulled a number of magazines out of his jacket pocket and with quick, jerky movements stashed the magazines beneath the counter where the ticket clock sat.

Marvin went on, "Then he changed into his red attendant's jacket. Wham, I'm at his side in a second. Surprised the hell out of him. I lifted him by the scruff of the collar, ready to smash his weasel face. Goddamn it, the son-of-a-bitch was light. By God, when I looked at that puny excuse of a man, skinny legs beating like a toy whirlybird, my fist only grazed him. I dropped the bastard." Marvin took a deep gulp from a bottle of water. He swirled it around in his mouth, as if he were trying to rinse out the dirty memory. "I spit—no, not at him, on the ground. Walked off. A car drove up, and Detective Graber and a cop jumped out and walked toward the guy. He started to run. I blocked him. We scuffled. Detective Graber reached for the handcuffs, clasped them on the guy and off they went."

"I hope I don't make a pest of myself?" Marilyn Graber smiled, as she entered the house. Then she caught sight of Marvin and wagged her finger. "You! You could have caused a major problem this morning. It's up to the police and the court to—"

"Sorry. I know, I know," Marvin said, raising both hands. "For a moment it felt good. If he had been bigger, believe me I would have hurt the bastard."

"The case is getting more complicated. We confiscated a large stack of magazines hidden in his booth dealing with homosexual pedophilia." She turned toward me. "I don't know where they photograph this stuff.. . .Ugh. Of course he denied they're his."

Marvin shouted, "Oho! To this I can be a witness. I was watching him when he took some mags out of his jacket and stashed them below the ticket clock."

"Ah! That's where we found them. Your surprise visit was good for something after all." She smiled. But her smile was not a happy smile. "We believe that he indeed thought Stephanie was a boy."

I suddenly remembered the attendant's first outcries of denial to me. He had kept repeating *he* rather than *she*. I had attributed this to poor English.

Marilyn Graber went on. "That's what we think he was after. A boy. Now," she held up her hand to ward off Marvin's questions, "I came across a year-old file, before I joined the Beverly Hills Police Force." Marilyn proceeded to tell us about a horrific case where a little boy was molested in the men's room of the gas station next to the toy store. Those parents had dropped the case on the advice of the child's psychiatrist.

Marilyn checked out the attendant and learned that he had worked at the parking lot a year ago. She was convinced that this attendant and the molester were one and the same person. She tried to influence us to prosecute, to take this man off the streets. "In the interest of other children," as she put it.

A few days later, I was at the Frostig Center. I was attending a meeting with a group of women who had elected me president of the auxiliary, Learn and Return, that raised funds for the Frostig Center. The door opened, and one of Stephanie's teachers, Trudy, motioned me to follow her. Within seconds we were running toward the playground. Breathless, Trudy explained, "Steffi had a fight with Erik. She's never like this. Has anything happened to upset her?"

I briefly summarized the "incident" with *the man* to Trudy. The fight now made sense to her. Stephanie had hinted to her classmates about a *man* and a dollar.

Trudy slowed down and lowered her voice. "Erik shoved a quarter at her, demanding she pull down her panties. Stephanie flew into a rage. She's usually so mild mannered." Trudy shook her head. "Can you imagine, she threw herself at him, tore his hair. . .punched him. Then he bit her and threw her to the ground."

We arrived at the playground as ten-year-old Erik was being dragged off to the principal's office. Stephanie burst into tears and ran to me.

She sobbed. "Erik! That—" She paused, perhaps searching for a suitable expletive to use in front of her mother. "He said I was a bad girl. To take money. . . and that's what *he* wanted me to do!" Her face was wet and red, and she cried so hard she couldn't stop shaking. "I threw his quarter at him! I hate him, hate him. I'm *not* a bad girl."

Before going to sleep I told Marvin the story with Erik. His breath came heavy. Then I told him about the appointment I had made with the district attorney.

"It's tomorrow, at 3:30; I hope you can make it?"

"You might have phoned the office while I had a calendar in front of me, but then, you seem quite set on handling this entire matter yourself."

"I tried reaching you all afternoon. Where were you anyway? You said you wanted that guy locked up. Don't we agree on that?"

"You made an appointment to see the DA with or without me." He withdrew to the far side of the bed.

"Marvin," I said. "That's the time he gave me. We both need to talk to the DA as soon as possible. You know they have to let the guy go if we don't prosecute." Marvin's back remained rigid. "Marv," I tried to break the silence. "This entire thing. . .I want to get it over with, don't you?"

"You were going to see him with or without me."

"Yes." I was surprised at how sharp my voice sounded. "That is the time he gave me. You are quite right."

"I'll be there. Don't you worry. One of us has to keep a cool head."

Our harsh words kept me awake. If we had been on a teeter-totter, we both would have noticed the shift in our balancing act.

Stephanie and I arrived at the courthouse half an hour early. Stephanie had been reluctant to dress in the jeans and patterned shirt she wore on the day of *the man*. Before entering the building, I pulled a hairbrush from my purse to smooth her hair.

"Stop it, Mom. I hate it when you do this. Especially right here on the street."

"You want to look presentable, don't you?"

"Whatever. I hate my hair. I hate these dumb pants. The whole outfit makes me want to puke."

I pulled her by the hand as I crossed the street, held the large doors open for her, and marched her to the elevator. "Sorry, Pumpkin. You had to wear—"

"Yeah, yeah, yeah. What I wore that day. I know. I'm sick of the whole thing." Suddenly she grabbed me. "Mommy, does the DA have a gun?"

"I don't think so. The DA is a lawyer, like your father. Did the gun in Detective Graber's purse scare you?"

"No. She's my friend. Mom, I'm afraid of this DA!"

"Sweetheart—" I broke off as the elevator arrived. "He's on your side." I continued, while riding to the fourth floor, "Like Marilyn. Now listen, the law is a complicated thing. You'll have to tell your story many, many times. But you have nothing to be afraid of. The law is here to protect us from people who are not well."

"Sick?"

"Yes. Like this man. He's really a sick man."

"I was sick. Three years ago."

I hugged her. "Pumpkin, not that kind of sick."

"I know. He's sick in the head. Daddy said he's crazy, *converted*."

I smiled. "*Perverted,* Stephanie. That means he turned away from the good and normal things in life. We have to see that he gets help and won't scare any other kids."

We sat outside the DA's office. Waiting. Stephanie shivered. "Is that man going to be here now?"

"No. He's in jail."

She snuggled close. "Mommy! I'm scared of that man."

I tightened my arms around her, wondering if we were doing the right thing.

Detective Graber strode down the hall and escorted us into the DA's office. Marvin arrived a few minutes later. He looked as if he had been in a hurry and left his jacket unbuttoned, which had partially crept off his shoulders, his tie hung askew. I smiled. He did not fit the stereotypical image of a successful attorney.

We answered the questions. Stephanie remained calm. The DA got down to specifics. "Is this the outfit she wore that day?"

"Yes," I said. "Exactly. Down to the shoes."

"Is it all right if I ask your daughter to open her pants for me?"

Marvin and I answered in unison. "It's all right."

"Now Stephanie, please take off the belt for me."

Stephanie struggled. She found it impossible. "You do it, Mommy."

"It's okay, honey," the district attorney said. And to Stephanie, who seemed reluctant, he said, "It's okay, honey. Now would you please open your pants for me." She tugged at the zipper, attempted to stand, but was told by the DA to remain seated. The zipper remained unzipped.

"Thank you. That's fine. Leave it be. Will you please wait outside for a few minutes while I talk with your parents?"

Marilyn Graber took Stephanie by the hand. "Come on, Steffi, I'll get us some Cokes, okay?"

The district attorney had formed his opinion quickly. "Your daughter is very believable," he said. "She's consistent in her story. I'll prosecute, even though a rape has not occurred. I feel this man is potentially dangerous." He dropped his pen on the table, and he stared past us through the window toward the Moorish-style tiled roof of the Beverly Hills City Hall. "I must warn you, the defense will pull every trick in the book. Whatever lawyer is appointed will use Stephanie's handicaps to the defense's advantage. They'll try to make her out to be an incompetent witness."

This is precisely what Marvin feared. Stephanie had a healthy self-image. What would happen if someone were to label her *retarded*? How would that affect her? I turned to Marvin for guidance. He sat absorbed in studying the cuticles of his fingernails.

"Why did you say he seems to be 'potentially' dangerous?" Marvin asked the District Attorney.

"This man. . .I feel there's something wrong here. He swears he didn't touch *him*. He's married, has a wife, three kids. Some latent homosexuals have problems admitting to themselves they are homosexual. They have trouble making the switch to a relationship with a consenting adult. So they get their kicks from molesting little boys." He looked at Marvin, then at me, his face a somber mask. "Sex offenders who act out of a distortion of their sexual orientation are potentially the more dangerous ones."

Marvin asked, "What exactly would it entail? The prosecution of this man?"

"First, there would be a preliminary hearing. The judge would hear both sides. Then the trial. The guy has no money, the court would appoint council for the defense."

Marvin shook his head, almost to himself he said, "And Stephanie?"

"You must know your own daughter. Whether she can handle this. She *is* believable. I told you that."

"Decisions," Marvin said, his breath hissing. "Sorry, we can't make our mind up on the spot." We shook the DA's hand in parting. "We'll be in touch."

"Please do," said the DA. "The guy can't make bail. A few more days and we'll have to file or let him go."

We were at the door. I turned. "One more thing. Does he know who we are?"

The DA shook his head in a definite *no*. The door closed behind us. Then the DA opened it again and called to us, "When it goes to court he'll know. He's got a right to know who his accusers are."

The next day Marvin had to fly to Sacramento. I watched him put yet another shirt into his overnight bag. "You're packing as if you're going away for days."

"Don't look so forlorn. And don't worry. I'll be back tomorrow night."

When I put Stephanie to bed that night, she whispered in a husky voice, "Mom, I asked some of my friends to spend the weekend. I asked Angela. She said her mother won't let her. Then I asked Patty; she couldn't come. And I hate Linda! She flat out said no!"

I was surprised. All of them were friends from the Frostig Center who'd spent nights at our house before. It occurred to me, this related to the incident with *the man*.

"Steffi, I'll talk to some of the mothers tomorrow. Now go to sleep and dream of fairies and angels." I kissed her and put the large Snoopy next to her bed. She sighed in contentment and soon the comforter floated up-and-down with her regular breathing.

She looked so peaceful, cuddling in her pillows. But suddenly, I saw her as if I were in a nightmare, the sight of her sleep-flushed face changed. Her face appeared behind the glass of the goldfish bowl, as I'd seen her in the doctor's office. Distorted. Her eyes were open and stared into space. They grew large and frightened, out of proportion with her face. Small orange fish swam in confusion over her cheeks, her nose, and her chin. I wanted to scream, the vision was so real. I shook my head rapidly, to bring myself back into the reality of Stephanie's bedroom, and saw my child sleeping peacefully in her white, eyelet-embroidered sheets.

But I was left with bewildering thoughts. Will a trial confuse her mind? Will it do harm to her self-image? Is it right for us to risk her growing self-awareness and perhaps hinder her progress?

My mind gave me no rest. I needed to talk with Marvin, but he was in Sacramento and had forgotten to leave the name and telephone number of the hotel. I went downstairs and prepared a hot cup of milk with honey, my usual remedy for raw nerves, but even that little tonic did not calm me.

When I finally went to bed, I was exhausted. Strange, how the clock and its beat echoes the rhythm of the human heart. Tick tock tick tock. The luminous dial showed the hour to be 1:30. I must get my sleep; I must get my sleep. But sleep would not come. My nerves attached themselves to the clock, to my heartbeat. Pulsing sounds of silence.

A car drove up the hill, turned onto our street, shut off the motor, and coasted to a stop. I heard a car door open, I heard it close. The ticking of the clock sped up, louder, louder, racing my heart.

The man. It must be *the man.* I jumped out of bed, crept to the window. And parting the drapes I peered down to the darkened street.

What I saw made me smile. A neighbor's teenage daughter lay curled within the arms of a young man on our front lawn. Smoke spiraled upward as they passed a cigarette from one to the other, their faces tilted toward the waning moon.

There were valid reasons why Linda didn't want to sleep over any more. She had her own problems, far, far worse than Stephanie's.

I learned about those troubles the night I went to the Rape Center, to hear a speech by a district attorney from New York. This DA's agenda was to convince the audience that *every case* should be brought to trial.

After the lecture, I rushed out of the hall and was surprised to collide with Doris, Linda's mother. We went to a coffee shop, and over a cup of soothing hot chocolate she confided Linda's story to me.

Doris had dropped her daughter off at a girlfriend's house to spend the night. Linda found it strange that the mother of this nice middle-class family was nowhere in sight. The girls prepared and ate their dinner of cereal and bananas.

Linda's nine-year-old girlfriend and her seven-year-old sister took Linda to their bedroom, where they begged her to play their father's games with them. If not, he would hurt them. Stub out cigarettes on them. Linda was horrified when they showed her their backs and buttocks covered with burn wounds. She was too scared to run away. Later, the father raped her.

When Doris found out, she went to the police and had the father arrested. After I heard Linda's story, Stephanie's incident with *the man* seemed a mere trifle, something not important enough to be pursued. Still I was torn between wanting to put *the man* behind bars and wanting to let him go and be able to forget the entire incident.

Several days later, Marvin stormed into the kitchen with Stephanie trailing behind, dragging a large purple poodle.

"Hey, did you have a good time, Steffi?" I asked her, "Did Daddy win this for you at the shooting gallery?" Then I noticed the large rip in Marvin's pants. "What happened to you? Did you fall?"

"That's part of the story. We were just at the DA's office—" He saw the question on my face and hurled these words at me. "I dropped the charges!"

"You what?" I couldn't breathe. "Without discussing it?"

"There's nothing to discuss. I knew you'd see it my way." He sucked in his lips, furrowed his brow in a lopsided way, looking like a kid who might get into trouble. "She's my child too."

"But why? Why?"

Then he told me what had happened at the Santa Monica pier.

Stephanie and Marvin had gone there to have fun, to spend a father and daughter afternoon, eating corn dogs and ice cream cones, riding on the carousel, and aiming for prizes at the shooting gallery. The two separated for a moment, while Marvin entered a phone booth to make a call. When he left the booth, Stephanie was nowhere in sight. Marvin ran to the parking lot. No Stephanie. Then he spotted a parking attendant, about the size of *the man*. Marvin, feeling a rush of adrenaline, ran, tripped, fell, ripped his pants (he pointed at his bloody knee when he came to that part in the story). The attendant was by now opening the car door for an elderly gentleman who was about to slide behind the steering wheel. At that point Marvin prepared to lunge at the attendant. The young man wheeled around, taking a martial arts defensive stance. Marvin froze. He saw the face bore no resemblance whatsoever to *the man*.

"Daddy, Daddy!" Stephanie came running across the parking lot, lugging the purple poodle. "What're you doing, Dad?"

The man still glowered. Marvin felt dazed. *Yeah, what the hell am I doing?* "Sorry," he said to the attendant, "I mistook you for someone else."

"Who?" Stephanie asked.

"Where have you been? I told you to wait for me by the phone booth."

"I'm sorry! Please don't shout, Daddy! I just walked across from you to the railing, to look at the people on the beach."

"Don't do that again. When I tell you to wait, you wait! On the same spot. . . till I get back. Understand?" He lifted up her chin, wiped her wet cheek. "Don't cry, Steffi. I thought that the—Never mind."

"You thought that *the man* had kidnapped me or something? Don't you remember? He's in jail, and this man doesn't look anything like *my creepo*."

She said the crucial words. When Stephanie called the man *my creepo*, something clicked. Marvin saw the distortions created by the attention given to this matter. He foresaw future problems. That's when he phoned the DA who was able to see him that same afternoon.

The two men reached an agreement quickly. Marvin let the DA know that he was willing to drop the case, but he wanted some sort of guarantee that other children would be protected from this molester. The DA suggested that he would enter into a plea bargain with *the man*, promise him immediate release in exchange for his voluntarily registering as a sexual offender—pedophile. This would lead to the protection of other children. The attendant would lose his job at that particular location and would not be able to work near children—such as a school, a park, a toy shop, or a children's clothing store. *The man's* fingerprints and his mug shot would go on record where they would be kept. If a reported crime fit his description, his identification and his modus operandi would be on file. Justice would be served.

Marvin came to the end of his story, leaned back in his chair, and breathed a deep sigh. "Now we can put this whole sordid affair behind us. The less we talk about it, the better for Stephanie." He got up, walked to the wet bar, unscrewed a bottle of J&B, and poured himself nearly a tumbler full over ice.

A few days later, I pulled up at the Frostig Center to pick up Stephanie. Linda's mother signaled me. "Our trial is coming up next Thursday," she said. "Want to come? Might prepare you for what you'll have to go through."

I felt guilty—as if I had let her down, and all other mothers in similar situations. I told her what happened and added that *the man* had been required to register as a pedophile.

"Oh," she said, her eyes avoiding mine. "That's all right then. Better for Steffi."

I didn't go to court when Linda's case came up. Later I learned that the jury found *that father*, who had committed those unspeakable deeds, to be of unsound mind. He was committed to the psychiatric ward of a state prison. He would only stand trial and be sentenced when, and after, he was judged to be mentally fit to stand trial.

Chapter Twelve

Miracles and Roses

Life to me is a gift. . .
—Stephanie Finell

Three years went by. They were turbulent years. Great American, the insurance company that Marvin, its CEO, had moved from New York to Los Angeles was sold by Eugene Klein, and the new owner relocated it to Cincinnati. When Marvin wrote his own ten-year contract, he cleverly stipulated that he would serve his term in the Los Angeles area only, knowing that Stephanie would need the schooling of the Frostig Center. When Great American relocated, Marvin was out of a job, and though we had the same income, he had too much time on his hands. He started the First Los Angeles Bank with friend and banker Joseph Digange and several lawyers, and a few years later he invested in an energy firm in Newport Beach. He bought a racehorse and spent much of his free time at the track.

Steven, after Treehaven in Arizona, had tried to adjust to our home life for a year and attended his old school, El Rodeo. Then he chose to go on a new adventure. For his freshman year in high school, he had selected New York Military Academy, for there—as *Boys Life* magazine promised—he could learn to fly.

But while Steven still lived at home, my mother kept interfering in our lives. She slipped Steven money, sabotaging our efforts to teach him how to budget his allowance and do his chores. "The poor boy" was her constant refrain, "You adopted him. Treat him with more love." *Adopted.* I wanted to scream at her, he is my son, *my* son. But she delighted in using that word: *Adopted.* As if to tell me, "He is no more yours than he is mine."

Mother could not wield her influence over Stephanie. There was no bribing her. Stephanie had a way of seeing through most people. She felt no need to play games.

Meanwhile, Celia had met a man who opened a butcher shop in Portland, Oregon, and left us to marry him. Her decision and departure came quite suddenly, and after she had spent so many years with us, she left a large void. Stephanie missed her terribly, whereas Steven had often been hostile toward her, sensing that she preferred Stephanie. There had been numerous occasions when I admonished her to treat Steven with more understanding, but she found this hard, especially as he grew older and more rebellious toward everyone—with the exception of Stephanie, toward whom he was aloof but always protective.

In the summer of 1977, Stephanie was thirteen and a half. She was growing into a young woman. Her hair had grown long since the time *the man* had called her a boy, and it curled in waves below her shoulders. She was wearing her first superfluous bra and began shaving her almost hairless legs. But while her body was maturing and going through hormonal changes, her learning ability remained that of a seven-year-old. I reasoned, after all, she *is* only seven years old, if we counted the years after her awakening from the coma.

In August, Stephanie and I left for Paris and Lourdes. Marvin was to meet us ten days later in Paris, and then the three of us would fly to Spain. Meanwhile, during our time in Europe, Marvin's parents invited Steven to accompany them on a Caribbean cruise.

Stephanie was still spatially disoriented and could not follow directions. I had to take her to the toilet in restaurants and accompany her to our room in hotels. At times she would feel sick to her stomach and throw up; other times she complained of violent headaches. I usually could tell if one of her *maladies* was coming on, as her face would suddenly drain of all color and she walked as if in a daze. These were symptoms we knew were related to the scarring in parts of her brain. She still had short-term memory loss. This dysfunction led her to try and find this or that, much like a blind person tapping through familiar rooms but not finding what they were searching for. She got easily frustrated when having to work through everyday activities, much like someone doing a jigsaw puzzle with many of the pieces missing. Only she didn't know what it was that was missing, while she kept looking for the nebulous to complete the picture.

I wasn't clear as to what I expected from the sacred waters of Saint Bernadette, but in Lourdes I secretly hoped a miracle would occur. Marvin was skeptical, but he didn't discourage us.

When we arrived in Lourdes, after having visited all the tourist must-sees in Paris, we found that the hotel had mixed up our reservation. We were listed for September, and it was still August, the month of travel for French city dwellers. This hotel, like most hotels in Lourdes, was fully booked. But Stephanie rescued the day. With a disarming smile and her head inclined, quite unaware of her charm as her shoulder-long hair curled to one side, she addressed the fortyish owner, "*Monsieur*, this is a place for miracles, *Oui?* Will you not make a teensy-weensy miracle and find a room for us?"

What could he do? His comma-like mustaches bobbed up and down, and he flirted with her and suggested we first have lunch, compliments of the hotel. He was impressed when he watched the American *petite fille* relishing frog legs and spearing some of my garlic-butter-dripping snails onto her fork. After searching through his reservations again, the owner miraculously found a spacious room with eight beds for us, albeit beneath the mansard roof. He apologized for the dormitory style accommodation, which he explained, would normally be occupied by a group of nuns. We found it charming with its slanted ceiling. Stephanie, like Goldilocks, jumped from bed to bed to test them out (no, there were no bears expected in this room)—and as a bonus, being so high up, we had the best view in the hotel.

Beyond the slate-tiled roofs of the city, beyond the plane and poplar trees, we could see the gray ribbon of the River Gave winding its way through emerald meadows. At night we sat on the high windowsill and watched torchlight processions in the ever-present drizzle marching along the river beneath forests of umbrellas. The torchlights' mirror images flickered like orange flames in dark waters.

The sun was gilding dew-wet roofs when we awoke, but soon it hid again behind a layer of thick clouds. I hoped for a miracle for Stephanie, but I had read enough to know that the spontaneous healing miracles occurring here at Lourdes usually related to diseases of a metaphysical origin, and Stephanie's case was different. Her brain was damaged by scars. There was no autoimmune system that could suddenly right itself, no cancer cells that could spontaneously stop dividing. My prayers were modest. I prayed that Stephanie would remain seizure-free. I prayed for a miracle that would improve her short-term memory. I prayed for improvement in the use of her right hand and arm. I prayed that her sense of direction would get better. I hoped and prayed that Stephanie would be able to get married, give birth to a child, and live a productive life.

When we walked to the baths to be immersed in the sacred waters, I was surprised to witness a small miracle in Stephanie. Normally, she was restless, but now she stood patiently in queue for several hours. Ever observant, she pointed to the men's shorter line, saying, "Mom, not so many men believe in miracles. Not like women. If we were men we wouldn't have to wait so long."

The two of us, plus four women pilgrims, undressed in a small antechamber. Two nuns in blue habits sped up the shedding of clothes, no dawdling allowed. They snatched our garments and hung them on wooden pegs. The white-gray marble floor chilled our bare feet. The nuns worked efficiently, and once our clothes were off we found ourselves wrapped in blue cotton sheets. Stephanie was the first to enter the cubicle of the sunken square marble tub. The water looked murky. Stephanie stepped back. One of the nuns grabbed her by the wrist, dragged her to the tub, then flung her into the water. Stephanie stiffened, resisted. The nun pushed, and down and under she went. Then she came up spitting water and—she smiled! "Brrr, its cold," she said.

I was next. It was the middle of August, the warmest month in summer, but the water felt as if it had come from a glacier. The immersion was short, and moments later we found ourselves back in that same chamber, shivering and dripping wet.

I helped Stephanie with her clothes. No one had advised us to bring a towel. The blue sheets the nuns had provided by then were soaked and helped little to dry us. It wasn't easy to pull jeans up on a wet body. Finally Stephanie was dressed and stepped outside to wait for me.

The drizzle had turned into a light rain. When I finished dressing and closed the door behind me, I found Stephanie standing beneath the overhang of the roof next to the rotund priest who for hours by now had been reciting the "Hail Mary" into his microphone, in French, Spanish, and Italian. There she stood, on the wooden platform, wearing her red slicker, its hood pulled up over her wet hair. The priest in his brown cowl stood next to Stephanie, pushing the microphone toward her while addressing the crowd. "*Et maintenant, notre petite fille des Etats-Unis va réciter un « Je vous salue, Marie » en anglais.*"

Oh my God, he's telling the people that Stephanie will recite the "Hail Mary" in English. Stephanie responded with a hearty, "Amen!"

"*Non. . .non. . .non. . .*" The priest fluttered his arms and hands like an excited mother bird, and looking at me, he pointed to Stephanie with his thumb. "The 'Hail Mary,' the 'Hail Mary,' tell her to say it in *Eenglish!*"

"She doesn't know the 'Hail Mary.' We're not Catholic." I tried to explain to the flabbergasted man of God.

I can still picture his eyes. The whites getting whiter around their brown irises, their expression growing from bewildered to incredulous. He probably thought, *What, not Catholic? Why are they here*?

I answered his unspoken question, "But we do believe in miracles!"

Stephanie took my hand, and when we walked back to our hotel, many in the throng of waiting people clapped when Stephanie passed and awarded her a *Bravo!* and a smile.

We felt a sadness leaving Lourdes the following afternoon. We met Marvin in Paris and flew to Madrid. Here in a *tasca,* one of the many charming small tapas bars in the city, a handsome young man sent Stephanie a red rose—her first—much to the chagrin of Marvin, whose impulse was to send it back. I tried to explain to him, who seemed oblivious to the fact that his little girl was growing into an attractive young woman, that the polite thing to do was to smile and accept the flower.

Marvin and I loved flamenco, and we had taken Stephanie to several performances in Los Angeles. Stephanie too had come to love the dance. Sarah, Marvin's former secretary, now lived in Madrid to continue her study of flamenco.

We visited the school where some of the famous flamenco dancers taught. Later, we all went out to lunch with Paco, Sarah's friend and mentor. The sky was unseasonable gray, and a heavy drizzle wet us, while the cobblestones glistened, polished by the rain. Paco began to dance, humming, "Singing in the Rain." He took Stephanie by the hand and soon the two were dancing down the street. Then he clapped his hands, stamped his feet, and in a husky voice sang a *bulería*. Stephanie copied his steps and clapped her hands, all in good rhythm.

I thank Stephanie for that memory, dancing flamenco in the rain, on a cobblestone street in Spain.

> I spoke to the Lord
>
> I said, please
> Let me know
> Who I am
> What I can do.
> Please Lord
> Let me know if I can do
> Anything.
> Anything well.
> Let me find something
> Let me choose something
> Good for me.
> You are the power
> You are the earth
> You are the sky.
> You are the Darkness
> And You are the Light
> And, I LOVE YOU.
>
> —Stephanie Finell, April 1986

Chapter Thirteen

Pressures, Explosions

Summer 1979

Stephanie's health had steadily improved. She had been seizure free for more than four years, and the doctors took her off her anticonvulsant medicines. It came quite suddenly when, in May 1979, Stephanie, now fifteen and a half, again began to suffer from minor seizures. The doctors put her on the drug Mebaral.

A few years earlier, when he was eleven, Steven had visited Spain and Germany with me. Stephanie stayed home with her father. When he was twelve, I took him on a two-week camping and horse-riding trip through the Cascade Mountains in Washington state, up to the Canadian border. I tried to fill the role of a father, for Marvin was not a man who liked roughing it when traveling and liked horses only when he could bet on them.

We had lived through several turbulent years with Steven. Now, in 1979, he was enrolled in Ojai Valley School. In this small town seventy miles north of Los Angeles, artists and seekers of spiritual truths had found refuge from the pressures and superficialities of Los Angeles and other large cities. The school reflected the atmosphere of the town and was located in a rural area. Steven had his own horse to take care of and loved riding in the hills. We visited him every second weekend.

Now, three months after Stephanie's minor seizures began, in August, all four of us were on a plane bound for Chattanooga to attend their cousin Scott's wedding. We told Stephanie she would not see Bud, Scott's father and her favorite uncle, until the actual wedding ceremony. He and Farol were getting a divorce.

Thinking about this in the plane worried her. She asked, "Won't Uncle Bud be my uncle anymore?" Before I could answer, she grabbed my arm, and with her teeth chattering, she whispered, "Mommy, I'm so cold, so cold—"

I held her, rang the stewardess for a blanket, scared that a seizure might follow. The cabin attendant reluctantly brought a blanket. Again I had to trouble the unwilling stewardess for a glass of water, trying to get Stephanie to swallow her Mebaral. Then the shaking began. A full seizure. *Oh please God, make it stop; calm her, please. Let the Mebaral work.* I held her tight, stroked her gently, and gradually the jolting movements slowed and finally subsided.

"Mom, I'm afraid. . .I'm so afraid," she murmured as she drifted off to sleep.

I was terrified. What was happening? Stephanie was going to be sixteen in three months. She was growing into a young woman. Were the seizures this time a manifestation of fear of the future—fear expressing itself metaphorically through the involuntary shaking and trembling of the body?

Marvin's parents were at the airport to greet us. Stephanie, still drowsy from the Mebaral, tottered down the landing steps to the tarmac. I would have liked for us to cancel all plans immediately and board a return flight, but with the entire family assembled in Chattanooga for the wedding, I did not follow my impulse.

At Farol's house, Stephanie met one of the house guests, a seventeen-year-old boy from New York. Jed looked like a blue-eyed Italian. Sensuous lips. Handsome. He flirted with Stephanie and she fell in love.

"Mom, do you think I'll ever get married? Do you think I can find a handsome guy to marry me?"

"Yes, Stephanie. When the time comes."

Stephanie didn't let Jed out of her sight. Later, we all went to see a movie in Farol's screening room. Jed was seated between Stephanie and her cousin Tracy when the boy put his arm around Stephanie's shoulders. When he glanced at her, I saw tenderness in his eyes. But when the lights dimmed, he turned toward Tracy and proceeded with some serious necking. Steffi nudged me and whispered she would like to leave.

That evening, Stephanie and I swam in Farol's pond-like indoor pool. A glass wall separated it from the living room, but despite the partition, it appeared to be part of the living area. We stepped into the water, the scene quite unreal, making me feel as if we were on a movie set. Water cascaded over rock walls where cattleyas and ferns grew in niches and fissures, while the moon, visible through a pointed triangle of glass—the roof—spilled a river of silver onto the dark green water.

Stephanie began to play. She swam in circles and did backward somersaults, which we called her sea-otter flip. Then we both held our breath and swam underwater, turning onto our backs, gazing at the moon through seven feet of water from the bottom of the pool. The liquid prism of water made the moon appear broken—as in a cubist painting—into many radiating and interlocking circles. We came up for air and swam to the rock wall, where we observed the moon from behind the curtain of water, a falling moon now, a sparkling arc of mother-of-pearl. Stephanie thrilled to the magic of water, the magic of the moon, the magic of the night, and she seemed to have forgotten her sadness over Jed.

After three days in Chattanooga, we were bound for the Florida Keys, where Marvin hoped to catch game fish in the Gulf's warm waters. I wanted to return to Los Angeles, but Marvin convinced me it would be good for the four of us as a family to take a mini vacation in Florida.

Perhaps he hoped to get closer to Steven when the two would go deep-sea fishing without Stephanie and me. I don't know what the reasoning was, but off to Florida we flew, even though Stephanie had suffered additional minor seizures in Chattanooga. But on the plane to Miami, she convulsed as she had years ago. In contrast to the stewardess on the earlier flight, the young woman on Delta Air couldn't do enough for her. She brought extra blankets and anticipated my need for a glass of water, bringing it before I asked for it. Stephanie shook her head when her lunch tray was brought and fell asleep with my arm around her after the medicine took effect.

We arrived at the Cheeca Lodge in Islamorada, in the Florida Keys, not quite midpoint between Homestead, still on the mainland, and Key West. During dinner in the formal dining room Stephanie began to seizure again. She didn't fall unconscious but was aware of the terrible shaking she couldn't control and aware of the other diners' stares. After the convulsing subsided, with my arms still around her, I tried to get out of my chair. She clung to me, buried her head in my chest, weeping, asking me to please take her to bed. That was exactly what I was planning to do.

I called Dr. Podosin in Los Angeles. "Give her an additional Mebaral, or two. It won't hurt her," he said.

Stephanie awoke in a happy mood the next morning, and after discussing it with Marvin, I decided to take Steven with me while I visited Lignum Vitae, a small island and a nature preserve. I had been commissioned to write an article about the island for the German geographic and literary magazine *MERIAN*. I felt that for half a day Stephanie would be in good hands with her father. And if she felt even better the following day, Marvin and Steven could go fishing.

When Steven and I returned, we found Stephanie asleep. Her breath came shallow, and she looked almost white. It was a comatose-like sleep, caused by the triple dose of Mebaral Dr. Podosin had recommended over the phone. Stephanie by now was falling (that's what it seemed like, a *falling*) from a convulsion into a deep sleep; then, after she awakened, she would stay in a state of awareness for only a few minutes before she convulsed again. She had not eaten since the previous day in Chattanooga and appeared weak. Marvin told me he had called Farol and told her about Stephanie's continued convulsions. He confided our predicament to her. To hospitalize Steff in Florida was one option;

however, none of the doctors in Florida were familiar with her particular medical history. We did not know how long we would have to stay in Florida with her, but to fly home on a commercial airline in her condition was impossible.

Farol asked Bud to help out.

Stephanie's dear Uncle Bud, in the midst of his divorce from Farol, acted like a true knight of yore. But this modern-day knight did not arrive on a white charger; rather he sent us his private jet to fly all of us back to Los Angeles. This was in 1979, when a there was a severe gasoline crisis. Bud himself had used his plane only in rare circumstances when he had to be in a place on business where no commercial plane could take him.

We were told the plane would pick us up in Marathon, in the Keys, the next morning, at 7:00 a.m. sharp. The alarm at 5:00 a.m. rescued me from a nightmare in which my child was convulsing, but when I entered Stephanie's room, I found myself in the same nightmare, a reality-based continuation of the night's terror. Stephanie was shaking more violently than ever in recent years, in the midst of a grand mal. We had to get her back to Dr. Podosin as quickly as possible.

She was weakened after a seizure and normally should have slept, but we had to dress her and meet the plane.

It was 6:15 a.m. I grabbed a cup of coffee and gulped it down. It burned my throat but cleared my head. We walked Stephanie to the rental car. A heavy tropical rain was pouring down and thunder roared in the darkened sky. Trembling in fear for my child's life, I had the absurd thought, *Is God a movie director? Are we the actors in an old-fashioned B picture? Why is it always thundering and lightning when Stephanie's life is in peril?*

Stephanie's extreme condition affected Marvin to such a degree he was too nervous to drive. He asked Steven, a good driver at sixteen, with his first driver's license in his wallet, to take the wheel.

The sky cleared. We passed a dazzling theatrical view of an orange sun, rising from the water, while purple clouds swirled above tourmaline mangrove islands, growing ever smaller in the rearview mirror. I craned my head to look at the spectacle. Stephanie, on my lap, lifted her head and looked back, and I could read in her shimmering eyes that she too was aware of that wondrous moment. Then her head rolled onto my shoulder, and she drifted off to sleep.

Steven noticed a police car pulling out from behind a billboard. "Damn—Dad! There's a cop following me."

"Slow down, slow down."

Steven slowed to 50 MPH, the posted speed limit. Suddenly the sirens screamed, and the blue light on the patrol car flashed. Steven pulled over.

"You were driving eighty-seven, young man."

"Officer," Steven said, "I have a very sick sister here. I was driving. . .at most perhaps sixty-five."

"Let me see your driver's license. California? Hmm, I clocked you at eighty-seven. Then you slowed down."

Stephanie started to convulse again.

"Please officer, my child—" I sobbed

Marvin interrupted and pointed to the flashing strobe light. "Turn off that flashing light," he yelled, "I have a sick—"

"My business here is with your son."

Marvin gestured toward Stephanie. "I have a convulsing child here, your goddamn flashes induce seizures," he screamed. "Turn it off, I tell you."

The police officer turned off the strobe.

Marvin calmed down and continued in Steven's defense. "I beg your pardon, officer, but my son didn't drive that fast. I would have told him to slow down."

The man of the law stood unmoved. "My business here is with your son."

Stephanie continued to convulse. "Officer," I pointed to Stephanie, "I have no water and she needs her medicine. Please, show a heart, she is very ill, please—"

I broke down crying. I pleaded again, pointing to Steff, "We have a plane to catch. I need water to give her a pill. My daughter is gravely ill, please. . .can't you see?"

Now he understood, but he still showed no mercy. "So that's why you were speeding, eh?" He began writing on his pad. For a moment he stopped and his thick and curved pink thumb pointed to the direction from which we had come." There's a good hospital in Homestead, or does it have to be Ca-li-for-nia, eh?" Now he shook his head, smiling mockingly, and writing. Writing slowly. His derision of California was clear. Sneering, holding us up while Stephanie shook and moved her arms wildly on my lap. I couldn't even jump out of the car and pummel him with my fists. I now understood, that in some cases, citizens were driven to attack the "upholder of the law."

"Officer, please, my son doesn't deserve this ticket," Marvin said. "You heard my wife, our daughter is very, very ill. The plane's waiting. . .we've got to. . .she needs. . ." Marvin shook, coughed, with a rasping voice he pleaded, "We've got to get her to the hospital and her doctor. Please, if you're going to write a ticket, put my name on it." He handed the police officer his license.

No use. The cop stood pillar-like, scribbling, ignoring us. It seemed to me as if he deliberately took his time. I wanted to strangle him. And Stephanie shook in my arms. Finally he finished, handed the paper to Steven who didn't want to sign, but Marvin told him to do so.

The plane had just finished fueling up when we arrived.

Stephanie needed to go to the toilet. Marvin couldn't come into the ladies' room with us, and I had to practically carry her, which was not easy, since she was five feet six inches tall and weighed one hundred and twenty-five pounds.

Finally we were on the plane. I gave her a pill now that we had water for her. A sofa, seating three, had been made into a bed. After laying her down John, the attendant and a former medic, secured Stephanie with a special seat belt. She snuggled under blankets, and her head rested on a fluffy pillow. Seizures continued to shake her, followed by periods of sleep. John observed Stephanie. His mouth curved in a half smile, and I saw tears forming in his eyes.

"A few hours ago I kissed my little girl in her crib, asleep, like Stephanie now. I guess even when they're older, you still see them as your little girl."

I watched Marvin swallowing hard, watched his Adam's apple bob, and I knew he was feeling the terror of her renewed seizures as acutely as I was.

As we neared the L.A. basin, the pilot radioed for a limo. We arrived at Dr. Podosin's office—as previously arranged—only to find the door locked, and a note advising us he could be found in the restaurant on the first floor of the building. Stephanie collapsed onto the carpet in front of the office, convulsing. People getting on and off the elevator stared, as I knelt next to my daughter, cradling her shaking body.

Marvin raced down to the restaurant. He found the doctor buttering a roll. "Doctor, Stephanie is lying in front of your door, convulsing!" Within moments Dr. Podosin and Marvin reached us.

"I'll put her in Westside hospital. The children's wing," the doctor said.

"Children's wing? She's almost sixteen."

"It's all arranged, I have other patients there."

I did not like this. I liked the way they had treated her at Cedars in the past. Getting her admitted was painfully slow. She couldn't walk. Two young men charged past us, wearing blue jeans, their hair wild. I overheard one of them mumble, "Stephanie."

"Are they doctors?"

"No way," Marvin said.

They were doctors, interns, and now they seemed to be in charge. Stephanie was put into a wheelchair and we followed her up into intensive care. Again we had to answer interminable questions.

We learned too late that Dr. Podosin had left her in the care of a colleague while he was on his way to a medical conference in Santa Cruz. He called us from the airport and tried to put us at ease by reporting that he'd seen Stephanie after she was in her room and that she'd appeared calm.

On our visit that night, we found Stephanie incoherent. She fell into a deep sleep while we sat by her bed, despite the bright ceiling lights shining into her face.

We returned the following morning and were told she was in the EEG room. The EEG showed normal brain activity, and an intern let us know that Stephanie would be discharged the next day. There had been no tests, other than measuring the amount of medication in her blood. A young intern, interested in psychology, believed her convulsions were a type of Freudian manifestation. A report stated that Stephanie had been seizure-free during the night. A heavy weight lifted off my chest. Then, a few minutes after having spoken with the interns in the hallway, I entered Stephanie's room and once again she was convulsing. I overheard a nurse by her bed saying, "Now, come on! What's the matter with you? What you're doing?"

"Can't you see? She's convulsing," I screamed at the nurse. "For heaven's sake! Don't you know what a seizure looks like?"

I ran to fetch the young doctor. "Come, you must see this, Stephanie is convulsing, badly." I grabbed him by the sleeve and dragged him down the hall toward Stephanie's room. "No wonder you said she had no seizures! The nurse standing right by her bed didn't recognize her convulsion. If she can't diagnose it, she obviously wouldn't chart it."

Nothing changed. Stephanie continued to have seizures and was doped up from medications. Marvin and I wanted to take her home.

We visited her at noon the next day. Her bed linens were soiled—showing stains of food—indicating she had not been assisted with eating. Her hair was matted and tangled. The nurses were busy with the younger children; no one seemed to have time for Stephanie. We had hoped that once in the hospital the doctors would try out different types of anticonvulsant drugs to bring the seizures under control. But this had not happened.

The report stating she'd had no further seizures was false—as false as the report saying she was alert. Stephanie was semiconscious, a condition she would later recognize and call "out of it." We wanted Stephanie to be out of *there*, and we got her dressed to take her home. We decided that if need be, and Dr. Podosin was still out of town, we would have her admitted to Cedars by another doctor.

No one brought a wheelchair for her. After a fifteen-minute wait, and still no sign of the nurse who promised to bring us one, I grabbed a wheelchair I'd spotted far down the hallway. But it lacked footrests. Stephanie's feet dangled and, scraping on the floor, kept stopping the chair. There was no one to escort us to the parking lot. We finally reached the car and took her home. A groggy Stephanie. She slept from midday until 7:00 p.m., looking dazed when she woke up. At the dinner table she ate two spoonfuls of applesauce. By now she looked quite thin and had probably lost ten pounds since the wedding in Chattanooga.

Stephanie's seizures were different now. At times she called out, "Mommy!" and, like a sleepwalker, came toward me with arms outstretched. Then she stiffened, followed by a grimace of the face, a spasm. Not the all-over shaking as before. I would tell her, "Relax. Nothing bad will happen to you, Pumpkin. Lie down. Calm, relax." Then I would stroke her and hum a melody to her, and slowly the seizure would pass.

I was glad we had not disconnected the intercom after Stephanie's earlier recovery. Now, years later, I again left it on at night and could be at peace when I heard Stephanie breathing rhythmically in her room.

A few days went by, and Stephanie kept having seizures. She fell asleep at the table after eating a grilled-cheese sandwich with a side order of pills. I phoned all morning trying to find someone who would admit her to Cedars, but since Dr. Podosin was her primary neurologist, we were told to wait for his return.

When Stephanie's life had hung in balance, I had been strong. But now, with these seizure episodes, not knowing what to do and where to get help, I was falling apart.

Marvin took my hand. I felt a surge of warmth. I clung to his hand, tanned, with strong square fingers, and tried to absorb some of his strength. He spoke gently, telling me that we'd weather this storm too.

Dr. Podosin came back from Santa Cruz and admitted her to the new Cedars-Sinai Medical Center. The atmosphere there was pleasant. Each room was a private room and immaculate. Stephanie had a pretty view. She told me she loved to look out at the hills and the Hollywood sign and watch palm trees sway in the breeze.

Again, all of her test results were "normal." Whatever storms were raging inside her brain remained hidden to all. No one could pinpoint the cause. The doctors at Cedars also believed the seizures were triggered by stress. We arranged for Stephanie to see a psychiatrist.

I wondered if Stephanie subconsciously worried about her future? What she would be able to accomplish in life, as she later wrote in one of her poems? *Please God, let me know anything, anything I can do well.*

Two months passed, and Stephanie had been seizure free. Completely. By late October, she had improved so much that Marvin and I decided it would be safe to take the two-week trip to China we had booked months ago. Stephanie's doctor was in accord and encouraged our trip, knowing we too were in dire need of a respite.

China beckoned. It had opened its borders to U.S. tourists a few months earlier. This year, 1979, we would have the opportunity to witness the awakening of the Red Giant, a time when China was still innocent of the influence of the West.

Steven was living with us again, and he seemed content going back to his old school in Beverly Hills. I wondered how he would behave once we were far from home. And I worried about leaving Stephanie at home with him. But then I reasoned, he loves his little sister, and he would act the responsible older brother and be protective of her. Yet in the back of my mind there were doubts. Could he be trusted? But Marvin too needed attention, and I thought a drastic change of scenery would be good for his increasing restlessness. Steven had been helpful around the house and spent time playing ball in the backyard with Stephanie, helping to enforce her eye-hand coordination. He played tennis three times a week at a friend's house half a block down the street from us, and I convinced myself that I could depend on him, and that he could be trusted.

Gloria, the timid Guatemalan housekeeper, who had followed Celia in our employ, could not assume the responsibility for Stephanie alone. We arranged for a young teacher from the Frostig Center to stay at our house, to supervise Stephanie and take her to and from school. But things got totally out of control.

When we were gone, Steven stopped going to Beverly Hills high school. He brought male and female friends to the house where they partied. They emptied the wet bar of its liquor. Telephone service between the United States and China did not work well in 1979. The teacher could not reach us, although the hotel telephone numbers were listed on our itinerary. Forbidding anything to Steven without an enforceable backup proved ineffective. After failing to reach us again in Canton (now Guangzhou), the teacher decided to take Stephanie home with her. Steven phoned my mother, who in turn called the police, telling them that the teacher attempted to kidnap her grandchild. She insisted the police tell this teacher to leave, she and Steven could take care of the house and Stephanie. Steven, who at sixteen stood over six foot two inches tall, looked mature for his age. Mother and the police arrived only minutes apart at our house. To the police, Steven appeared to be polite and reasonable. They believed the "man of the house," backed up by my mother. The teacher fled, Grandma stayed.

An urgent message left by the teacher awaited us in Hong Kong. We were shocked and tried everything in our power to get an earlier flight home, but all flights were overbooked, and it was impossible to change our schedule.

In the plane, homeward bound, Marvin ordered martini after martini, seeking temporary oblivion from what he would have to face. I popped an Empirin, when a migraine began gripping my head in its vise.

Chapter Fourteen

Sweet Sixteen

The taxi brought us to our house on Ridgedale Drive. Finally, we were home again. Stephanie's hugs and kisses almost made us forget our worries. Steven had wisely chosen to leave, hours earlier, and had taken refuge with my mother.

Stephanie must have sensed the tensions we had with Steven. She must have wondered about his sudden absence, but she never mentioned him, neither did she ask any questions. Not like in the plane when she worried, "Won't Uncle Bud be my uncle anymore?" None of this turmoil that affected Marvin and me so very much seemed to have any effect on her. I was afraid she'd suffer a seizure, but she stayed seizure free.

I was concerned about Steven and went to see him at my mother's home, but he kept his eyes to the floor and would not answer any of my questions. It was as if I were talking to a deaf-mute. He had been withdrawn at times before, but now he had erected a wall around himself, a wall that I could not scale.

I thought of the summer when Steven was four and a half years old, and he returned from a trip to his grandparents' house in Chattanooga. He had grown very pensive, and that night he called me to his room. Then he asked in a whisper, "Was I adopted, Mom?" He looked as if he might cry. Then he said, "What does adopted mean, anyway?" I shook my head in bewilderment when he surprised me with that question. He continued in his little voice, "Scott said I am adopted, like he and Tracy are."

I had tried to familiarize him with the word *adopted* early on, weaving the word into terms of endearment, calling him *my sweet adopted Schnooky-poo*, or *my very own adopted Sweetie -pie*. Now, I was suddenly wordless. Marvin and I had talked about the right words to use when the time came. "Let me get Dad and we will both talk to you about 'adopted.'" I ran downstairs to ask Marvin to come and help me explain the adoption issue to Steven.

When I neared the den, I heard his voice shout at the Monday night football game he was watching, "Goddammit, kill the bastard, stop him, stop him, oh noooooo—" I heard him throw his balled-up newspaper at the television. I hesitated.

I knew he'd had one too many beers (the only drink that appealed to him when he was watching football), and probably he had made too large a wager with his bookie, and at this stage in the second half of the game it looked as if he would lose the bet. I hated it when he was in this condition, which luckily did not occur very often. I squared my shoulders and confronted the raging bull—or lion, since he was a Leo. Our son was more important than his damn ballgame. Karin, get yourself together—I talked to myself—don't you start swearing too. Stay calm. This is an important time in our child's life and we should both be there to answer his question.

"Marvin, please come upstairs and help explain to Steven what adoption means. Scott told him that he is adopted, and Stephanie is not."

Marvin hardly looked up from the ball game as he shushed me away, hurling more obscenities at the television and shouted, "Damn that smart-alecky Scott. Go up. Go. . .go. You're a smart woman, you handle it."

I ran upstairs again, full of momentary anger, and full of love for our son, while trying to come up with an honest and caring answer.

When I returned to Steven's bedside, he had another question for me. "And Mom, what does it to mean to be a chosen child? Scott said we are special, we were chosen." "Chosen, Stevie? Is that what Scott said? Like going into a bakery and choosing from an assortment of small cakes?" I was going lightheaded, imagining cupcakes with faces like baby girls or baby boys all lined up in frilly paper doilies in the shape of cribs and couples walking past them to "choose" one or the other. I now got angry at Scott too. "Steven, to adopt a child is an important decision parents make. Babies are not chosen like going to a store and choosing a pair of shoes, rather, like in our case, an opportunity arose and we said *Yes*. A big, booming *Yes* to adopt you." Steven smiled at my words. "Well," he drew out his words, sounding unsure again, "he also said I'm one of *them*."

His words, echoing his older cousin, angered me again.

I put my arms around Steven and told him he was not one of "them," but one of "us." The four of us. I held him tight and told him his story. "We had wanted a baby very much, but it seemed as if we could not have one. Then we were lucky. Your Godfather, Sol, called us and told us about a baby boy born two weeks earlier. Sol knew the young girl through his law practice, who was in a hurry to find a good home for her baby. That baby was you. He said we could be parents the next day. Out of the blue—we would be parents. The girl was desperate to find a loving family for her child. She had wanted to keep the baby, but her stepfather, after two weeks of enduring a constantly crying child, threatened her, he would throw her and the baby out the very next day."

Steven hand flew to his opened mouth, "Oh no," he said. Then he thought for a while and added, "What a bad man. But, she'd give her baby away? Like that?"

"What could she do? She was still in high school, she had no money."

"She'd give me away without knowing you and all?"

"Yes, Steven. In private adoptions, the birthparents do not meet the adopting parents. Sol told her we were good people. It must have been very painful for her. She loved you very much. We stood behind a doorway while we were waiting for her to leave Dr. Dietrich's office, your first baby doctor. When she passed by, she was crying and looked terribly sad and kept looking back over her shoulder and at her empty arms."

Steven sat up in his bed, his eyes wide open, trying to understand all that I'd said. "Why did she have empty arms?"

"Steven, she had left you at Dr. Dietrich's office, and from there we would pick you up. That was the arrangement."

We were both silent for a moment.

"Go on," he said, as if I were reading him one of his adventure stories.

"Well, it was raining lightly, she wore a scarf tied around her head, and looked like a little wet rabbit. She was so young, I had the sudden urge to adopt her as well. When she disappeared around the corner, we went to Dr. Dietrich's office and found the cutest little baby boy with the bluest eyes and we picked you up."

"And that is my own story? I don't remember that."

"Of course you don't. You were only two weeks old."

Why isn't Marvin here to help me? I wanted to scream down to the den, "Marvin!" But I didn't. Instead I finished my story. "Yes, Stevie, that is the story of how you came to be our own little boy."

"Are you my mommy then, or. . .?" His question drifted off and he didn't finish the sentence.

"Yes. I am your mommy, and you are our very own sweet son. And I love you very much."

"And Stephanie? How come she's not adopted?"

"Now that I had you in my arms, I didn't want another baby. I had you. Then, by some strange chance I got pregnant and had Stephanie. That's why you are so close in age. It was you in a way that helped bring Steffi into the world."

He furrowed his four-and-a-half-year-old forehead and looked like a little old wise man. I don't know how much he understood of all of this. I hoped it didn't burden him to know.

Now I confronted Steven at my mother's house, and he had shut himself away. My thoughts again drifted back to those earlier years, when at times Steven was angry and screaming. Then I would take him to his room and sit down in his large red rocking-chair, and pulling him onto my lap I would rock him and sing to him, "Stevie is a good boy, a good boy, a good boy, Stevie is a good boy, as everybody knows." He would slowly calm down and put his arms around me and nestle his head on my shoulder.

He was such a sweet-looking child, and at times he could be immensely lovable, but in general he did not initiate affection. It had to be coaxed out of him. Marvin would have wanted to have Steven run up to him when he came home from work and hug him and act like Stephanie did, leaping into his arms and showering him with kisses—well, from Steven he expected a hug or two at best. He could not understand that boys acted so differently from girls. From early on these two males in our family seemed to be in opposition to one another—at loggerheads, as Marvin called it.

"Steven, please talk to your mother," my mother's pleading brought my thoughts back to the present. There stood Steven, six foot two inches tall, but there was no red rocking-chair to help make it all okay again.

We had to make a decision as to where Steven would live, since Marvin did not want him to return to our house. Living with my mother was not a permanent solution.

All of this pressed on my mind. Far-reaching decisions had to be made. While my brain was on "over-drive," Stephanie pointed to the stack of her "Sweet-Sixteen-Birthday Party" invitations, still on my desk, with her birthday only a week away.

Steven and the teacher had promised they would take care of the invitations. With the turmoil of the past week, they had not been touched. But now Steff and I finished them quickly. I addressed the envelopes, Stephanie inserted the colorful invitations, we both licked the stamps, and I took them to our post office in time to go out that same day.

Many of Stephanie's friends whom she had known since K-grade in El Rodeo, and whose friendship we had kept up with sporadically, plus friends from the Frostig Center and Mahri's ballet school, came and gyrated wildly at Dillon's Disco in Westwood, but only until 10:00 p.m., when the teeny-boppers of the under-eighteen crowd had to vacate the place.

Steven and my mother were not invited.

Stephanie looked lovely in a white crepe de chine dress, short and flouncy, with a delicate flower pattern of violet and raspberry red. Grosse-grain ribbons, of the same colors, were woven into the cornbraids of her hair, framing her face, while the rest of her hair hung loose in waves. When she wasn't dancing with the boys, she danced with her girlfriends, Hugi and Michelle, Evie and Carol. I stood on the side, observing her lithe body glide over the shiny parquet floor, watching her swirl from the arms of a boy in a dark shirt and pants to another one in jeans.

I viewed Stephanie's former classmates from El Rodeo with a certain envy. A few of them now participated in tennis tournaments or excelled in playing the piano. And Stephanie, who had played "Für Elise" at age seven, could not even move the fingers of her right hand coherently.

Then my eyes wandered to several of the girls from the Frostig Center. A few of them had been born with disabilities. And I felt grateful for Stephanie's progress, aware of her grace.

Stephanie seemed weightless. The slowly rotating lights made her appear green, red, blue, silver, and golden with happiness. When my eyes beheld her floating past me, I felt as if I were a clay jar, now being filled with radiance and warmth. I loved her so much it hurt. While dancing, she threw me a glance here and there, tossed me a kiss, and told me how grateful she was for having this party. Then she whispered in my ear, she missed her big bro.

Later, when Marvin and I were in bed, he pulled me close, whispering that we three must stick together. "Steven is out of our life. I'll never let him live in this house again."

"You can't do that! Steven is not even seventeen."

"He's on his own. We'll sell the house, move into the condo."

This took me by surprise. He had said the condo purchase was an investment. I thought Marvin loved our house and our garden as much as I did. I thought he loved our morning walks with mists filling the canyons, the cooing of mourning doves, the scampering of a deer.

I came to understand, that the entire globe had to revolve around Marvin Finell.

Chapter Fifteen

Shadow Play

Spring 1980

Steven and Stephanie were now respectively seventeen and sixteen. There were still tensions between father and son, but they were on speaking terms again. It had been a stormy year for Steven. While staying at my mother's, he had a run-in with the law, and his probation officer mandated him to live in a boarding situation at Vista Del Mar. We met with him and his therapists and counselors as a family. He asked to be Bar Mitzvah'd, even though he was four years older than the customary thirteen. He studied the Torah and learned Hebrew texts and had a ceremony followed by a fine party, and best of all for him, he received many presents. His grandparents arrived from Chattanooga for the occasion. He basked in their attention, and for a while he seemed to be feeling good about himself.

Stephanie wanted to be baptized.

A few weeks before Easter, I took Stephanie to St. Albans Episcopal church in Westwood, where we met with Father Norman. We could not have found a more welcoming cleric. He invited us to the rectory the following Wednesday, and after I explained to him about Stephanie's learning disabilities as well as her father's Jewish and my own Lutheran background, he assured me that Stephanie could learn by listening. He immediately sensed her trusting spirituality and promised that she would be baptized as soon as possible.

That Sunday arrived. My friends Betty and Phyllis, Stephanie's two godmothers, stood by the baptismal font with me while Father Norman sprinkled her with sacred water. At that exact moment, a squirrel ran through the transept of the church. I interpreted this little creature of the wild as a good omen.

Fall 1981

Our house had been on the market for a few months, though we were still in the midst of making major landscape changes to our garden. We planned to add a Jacuzzi, a goldfish pond, and a waterfall, and Marvin wanted to create more space around the pool by building a retaining wall to support earth and lawn. It saddened me that Marvin planned to sell the house and move to Century City, into the investment condo. As elegant and spacious as the condo was, it was an urban setting, and I loved nature and our garden. And now, this garden would become more of a Shangri-La than ever.

Then Marvin came home one day and declared, "I've come to the conclusion that I'd be very unhappy in a condo. We'll sell the condo and stay right here."

"Really?"

"Would I kid about a thing like that?"

"No! I love this house. Let's call the agent and take it off the market."

"Done," he said.

Life seemed to be under control again. Stephanie had been seizure free since early August 1979. She had not taken a single Mebaral for two years. After graduating high school in June, Steven lived in a "single" apartment that Marvin had helped him find. He was independent, drove his first car (a canary-yellow Pinto), and worked for a finance company. Marvin permitted Steven to come home to have dinner with us once a week, but he had not forgiven my mother for her constant interference and did not want her to visit us. Mother was content to have Stephanie and me visit her in Santa Monica. Life was—if not sweet—at least bearable again.

Well, not entirely so. Marvin was morose most of the time. He drank heavily, sometimes leaving our bed in the middle of night to go to his office (installed in Steven's former room) to pour himself another Scotch. I thought I knew my husband well and had in the past always been able to intuit what troubled him, but now I was confused about his apparent alienation and restlessness.

What caused his pain? At this time we had no problems with Steven. And Stephanie was doing better than ever, advancing in her ballet class, getting the best parts in plays put on at her new school, Clearview, the school she now attended following the Frostig Center. In fact just last week, Marvin had applauded enthusiastically until I thought his hands would drop off when Stephanie danced and sang the part of Maria in excerpts from *Westside Story*.

Then Steven fell in love. Each time he came to visit, he talked nonstop about Beth. We were eager to meet this paragon of beauty and charm, Beth. Christmas neared, and Marvin's parents and Farol were in town with Tracy. We had Christmas Eve reservations at Jimmy's elegant restaurant in Century City, and everyone looked forward to meeting Beth. She was young, Steven's age, a pretty girl with flowing brown hair and large doe eyes. The next afternoon Steven brought her to our house for the traditional turkey dinner. She shocked Gammy by wearing a tee-shirt with the slogan, Sex, Drugs and Rock&Roll emblazoned on her chest.

It turned out to be a strange dinner as the evening wore on. Marvin was absent in mind and, for a short time, present in body only. He hardly touched his food and then announced he needed to run an errand. I didn't understand. He left his family for an obscure errand on Christmas Day? I felt like a fool, since Christmas was an important holiday for my mother and me, but acting the polite daughter-in-law to Marvin's visiting parents, I had neglected my own mother by staying home. And now Marvin rudely left all of us, including his parents.

New Year's Eve arrived. Aunt Farol and Tracy were still in town, and we invited several of Stephanie's friends, among them Michelle and our former realtor's two sons, to a small party at our house to ring in the New Year. Again Marvin acted out of character. Where did his mind wander to? He certainly was not in the moment and with us. Suddenly, about an hour before midnight, he leapt to his feet, hollering, "Okay, Farol. I'm ready. If you want me to take you to the other party, we'll have to go now."

Farol rose and took his arm.

"You're going to another party, Dad?" Stephanie asked, shaking her head in disbelief.

"Farol, you never told us you were going somewhere else," I said. "Are you leaving too?" I asked Tracy.

Tracy shook her head and kept dancing with one of our young friends.

"You'll be back before midnight, won't you?" I asked Marvin.

"Sure, honey, you can depend on it."

He did not come back until dawn.

A few days into 1982 Beth, aged only eighteen, and Steven, two weeks short of nineteen, eloped to Las Vegas. Soon Beth got pregnant with a child expected late in November.

Stephanie was excited that she was going to be an aunt, but she didn't quite see her brother as a father. "Steven's going to be a dad? No kidding, Steven?"

"It'll help make him more responsible. Anyway, that's what I hope," I said.

Early March, 1982

After twenty-one years of an unusually happy marriage (or so I believed, living in fantasy land), I suspected something was wrong. Marvin had to go on business to Maui, Hawaii, and he took me along. In March, Hawaii-bound, and after three martinis and champagne had loosened Marvin's tongue, he unburdened himself and told me about his cousin Judith. They had started a love affair when Marvin attended a family reunion of his father's thirteen brothers last summer. "I'm so sorry, honey," he wept. "Why didn't you come to New York with me, why did you let me go to Uncle Bob's birthday party alone?"

"Marvin, you said yourself it would be a fast trip, and you would just as soon go by yourself. We had been bored to death with another 'thirteen brothers' birthday party at your parents' house, remember? You usually go by yourself on business trips to New York, why ask me on this one?"

One of the thirteen brothers in attendance was Judith's father. When Marvin and Judith danced, Farol observed them. She later suggested to Judith that she go and visit Marvin. She gave her his room number. Judith happily did and spent the night.

The tornado of this romance moved with incredible speed, churning us in its funnel. Judith's second husband died in a car crash in January 1981, and her affair with Marvin began in June. She sold her former husband's general store and their home in Bedford, Connecticut, soon thereafter, made arrangements with his other heirs, his daughters, and moved near us in August.

This confession explained Marvin's morose behavior. It explained his drinking, which had by now increased to a dangerous level. Earlier I had thought the need for drink related to his sorrow for having a brain-injured child, but now I found his ever-increasing alcoholism had more complex causes. So far Marvin had treated me with respect and love. He had a strongly developed sense of justice. I considered him to be a man with a conscience. His little inner voice, which raised its objections and tried to stop him from wrecking our marriage and his relationship to his children, this insistent little voice had to be silenced. Immersion in alcohol would do the job.

Marvin, his eyes full of tears, swore he loved me and he loved Stephanie. Above all, he wanted our little family to stay intact. He pleaded with me to forgive him, and to give him time until he found a way out. He told me the situation trapped him. He loved Judith too and was concerned for her fragile mental state were he to leave her. She threatened suicide. She had been hospitalized for having tried it several times before. He must find a psychiatrist to help her before he could break up with her. The ball was in my court now. Would I act the shrew and cuckolded wife and throw him out? Would I be understanding and give him time? My anguish was constant, but I agreed to give him time.

When we came back from Hawaii, it was nearly impossible for me to act as if nothing had happened. Stephanie often asked, "Why are you crying, Mom? Why are you so sad?"

I evaded a direct answer and put on a forced smile. But Stephanie was perceptive and sensed something was wrong. Terribly wrong. Her sadness and bewilderment made it more difficult for me to remain strong but also made it more imperative to keep up a facade.

Chapter Sixteen

Prisons

Spring 1982

I needed to get away from the house, from Marvin. I needed to think. I ran away and took Stephanie with me. We boarded a Lufthansa flight for Berlin. It was late in March and seeing the spread of golden forsythias when we landed at Berlin Tempelhof reminded me of my childhood. Briefly I managed to push thoughts of Marvin and his lover into the recesses of my mind.

We stayed with old friends who lived in my former neighborhood of Niko-lassee, an idyllic suburb near one of Berlin's many lakes, and my friends treated us like family. I enjoyed showing Stephanie where I spent my teenage years af-ter the war. I took her to the house where we had lived and where my grand-mother died. Stephanie had heard many stories of my beloved Oma, who had raised me during the war and postwar years since my mother was working. We visited Halensee, where I had experienced some horrific times at the end of the war when the Soviets conquered Berlin. Some of the events I witnessed trau-matized me for years after the war. I withheld these stories of rape and may-hem from Stephanie, afraid they might upset her. We went to Steglitz, the part of Berlin where Oma and Mother and I were bombed out. I told Stephanie the story of the apartment building in flames, when Mother ran back into the fire to save my little toy bear.

"Grandma did that?"

"Yes," I said. "It was horrible to see the stairwell afire, the building implod-ing, but in the last moment your grandma emerged from the flames holding my teddy bear and my grandmother's silver teapot." Stephanie stared at me, her eyes wide.

"Grandma did that? She was a hero, right? I'll never be nasty to her again."

On Sunday we dressed to visit my half brother, Wolfdieter, and his wife, Babs, in East Berlin. I knew Stephanie would never be able to learn history from books, and I tried to teach her in these situations. I don't know if she really grasped the significance that a large city like Berlin, the former (and now again) capital of Germany, was divided into four parts after the war ended. Each of the four Allies—the Americans, British, French, and Soviets—received one of the four parts. At that time, my little family had been lucky to find ourselves in the British sector, and a few months later we were able to move to the American sector of West Berlin. Whereas my father's family escaped from Silesia—where I was born—and reached Dresden, the part of Germany that later became part of Soviet-controlled East Germany, the DDR. The eldest of my three brothers had moved to East Berlin, to attend the Humboldt University. I found it difficult to explain the political complexities of the Cold War era to Stephanie, an American child-woman. It could make no sense to someone who had never known anything but freedom.

Wolfdieter and his wife both worked, and we could visit them only on a Sunday, their one full day off. We would cross the border at Checkpoint Charlie, where we would exchange our passports for a one-day pass, but we had to return and cross back into West Berlin before midnight.

Stephanie laughed, "Like Cinderella, Mom, or our taxi will turn into a pumpkin."

She thought of the day trip to East Berlin as others might regard a trip to an exotic land. East Berlin was anything but exotic to me. I had crossed the border several times in past years, but only because I wanted to see my brother who could not leave to visit me.

We could not visit my two younger half brothers, for they lived in Dresden, and for the rest of East Germany we needed visas that took four weeks to process. No visa was needed to cross the border for a day to East Berlin.

We dressed in a strange fashion before we left my friends' place. We each put on three pairs of pantyhose. Although light, the many layers of thin nylons made us feel like sausages stuffed into tight casings. In addition to the hose, I pulled on two sweaters. We carried chocolate bars with us, coffee and cigarettes, and small gifts of cosmetics. My brother and his wife did not smoke, but the cigarettes could be exchanged for items they needed, reminding me of the early postwar years in West Berlin.

Wolfdieter picked us up at Checkpoint Charlie, and when we arrived at their apartment, a beaming Stephanie raced past our hostess to where I indicated the bathroom was. Here she took off the layers of hose. I noted the astonished expressions on Wolfdieter's and Babs's faces as I too rushed past them, following Stephanie. Feeling comfortable and able to breathe again, we emerged, dangling the nylons before Babs's nose, which in itself explained our rude behavior. And only then did we finally hug and greet one another properly.

Dainty flowers blossomed on recently manufactured Dresden porcelain—Meissen was produced for export only—its colors harmonizing with a cloth embroidered in a pattern of cross-stitching. Crystal glasses stood waiting to be filled with wine. Daffodils bloomed in a vase. Wolfdieter brought out slivovitz, a Bohemian plum brandy, which was tasty but burned my throat as it slid down. Steffi sipped lemonade. I remembered my sister-in-law's culinary skills from a prior visit. On this day, the *Mittagsessen*, the big meal Germans consume around midday (in this modern age only on weekends), Babs served a lamb roast melting on the tongue. This was accompanied by fresh spring vegetables, mashed potatoes, and a creamy brown gravy—or deservedly called a sauce, delicate as it was. We washed all of this down with a delicious Hungarian wine. Thick, black steaming coffee followed the midday meal.

Babs smiled apologetically, "My oven is not big enough. I just now put the apple torte in."

All the while, Wolfdieter drank hard liquor, had wine with the meal, and brandy with his coffee. He planned to take us sightseeing after we finished our meal, but I worried aloud about his ability to drive after consuming so much alcohol. "Don't worry," he said, "the only thing left for East Germans to enjoy is alcohol." I imagined an entire nation functioning, or rather malfunctioning, under the influence.

With a full stomach and the aftertaste of delicious food on my tongue, I began to believe that the citizens of East Germany did not suffer from food shortages, as we so often thought they did. It was only later that Wolfdieter told me how Babs had purchased the meat from a butcher, miles from where they lived, and only with a connection through her sister. The fresh spinach and French beans were bartered from a neighbor who had a small garden plot and grew vegetables in his tiny greenhouse. Everything Babs served had cost her great effort to procure and had to be partially prepared the night before, so it could cook while my brother picked us up at Checkpoint Charlie.

Wolfdieter wanted to show his American niece some of the famous sights of East Berlin. He took us to the Brandenburg Gate. We had driven down the (formerly so grand) avenue Unter den Linden and parked to look up at the quadrille of horses crowning the former city gate.

We did not have much time to spend on Museum Island and went straight to the greatest of them all, the Pergamon Museum. Stephanie and I marveled at the Ishtar Gates from Babylon (now Iraq), still dazzling in their blue- and gold-glazed magnificence after twenty-five hundred years. Stephanie grew very quiet and held her breath at so much beauty and overwhelming grandeur. Then we followed the great marbled halls holding the Temple of Pergamon—and Wolfdieter explained to Stephanie how it had been disassembled in Asia Minor by the German archeologist Heinrich Schliemann and was shipped to Berlin where it was reassembled and put on display as one of the great treasures of Greek antiquity. The ancient wonders were all there—but visited by few, even on Sunday. The museum itself seemed disembodied. After the doors of the museum shut behind us, the shoddiness of the city beyond stood even more in crass contrast to where we had just been.

Wolfdieter looked at his watch, slapped Stephanie on the back, and said, "Time to go back and have some cake."

"Cake? Yum, we're going to have some cake?"

"Yes, it'll be out of the oven by now," he said.

The cake was indeed out of the oven and cooling on the balcony. The apple torte awaited us. A latticework of golden brown pastry strips crisscrossed the succulent fruit, now a glistening bed of caramelized apples and smelling of cinnamon and spices.

The dishes had been cleared. Crystal plates anticipated the torte. Coffee steamed in a porcelain coffeepot, and whipped cream billowed in a bowl. Stephanie helped herself to a large piece and was in heaven. I must admit, her mother did not lag far behind.

While Stephanie helped Babs to clean up, my brother took me on a walk through a nearby wood. We had walked here on an earlier visit with Marvin, before my brother was married. Marvin suggested he would try and help Wolfdieter escape to the West. We walked here because this was the only place where Wolfdieter could be sure he was not being overheard by the Stasi, the East German security police, similar to the Nazi Gestapo.

It was still the same dense little forest with thick ferns growing near a meandering stream. The wood reminded me of the Grunewald, the forest near where I grew up. For a moment I forgot I was in East Berlin, the shabbiness of the city was masked by verdant nature. The infamous wall was not in sight, and the lakes and woods that stretched from east to west tricked me into thinking the city was not divided but was as one.

The low afternoon sun slanted through the trees at an angle, gilding the branches, and a light breeze stirred the leaves into a many shaded dance of greens. Legions of frogs hopped and croaked on boulders in the sandy stream's bottom. I had told my brother about Marvin and his mistress cousin, and I mentioned that Stephanie did not know about our recent marital problem.

I pointed to the frogs and said, "My life is the reverse of the old fairytale. I kissed my prince and he has now turned into a frog."

My laugh sounded forced and hollow, and tears rolled down my cheeks. Trying to put levity into the situation did not help. Wolfdieter hugged me and told me to be patient, maybe Marvin would come to his senses.

Then he wrinkled his forehead in thought. "My God," Wolfdieter said. "They are as closely related as you and I. They share one set of grandparents together." I had not thought of that.

Back at the apartment, Babs and Stephanie had set the table for the evening meal, the *Abendbrot*—a lighter meal—with cold cuts and assorted breads.

We (not Stephanie) drank more of the white wine, more slivovitz, and when it came time to say goodbye to Babs, we were so stuffed we practically rolled down the stairs.

Wolfdieter made fun of his tiny Trabi, an ugly black box of a car officially named Trabant. Made in East Germany, it was a clumsy imitation of the Volkswagen. The wait—from the date of their application to purchase the car to the actual date when it became available for delivery—had been six long years.

Stephanie squeezed into the back seat. The Trabi sputtered and trembled. "Verdammt!" my brother cursed.

"Dammit," Steffi echoed. I agreed. Of all times: *Start car, start!* Our visitors' permit would run out in half an hour. Pumpkin time. The Trabi coughed, wheezed. The motor caught. Wolfdieter looked at me, his lips stretching into a grin. His arm went around my shoulder. I cradled my head in the crook of his neck and felt the flow of his sadness meeting my own.

When would I see him again?

"You'll make it in time."

The lump in my throat did not allow me to speak. I stroked the gift he'd placed into my hands as we left the apartment. I thought of our love for Bertolt Brecht, the great German playwright, a renowned Communist, who had chosen exile in the United States during the Nazi years but then, after the war, made his home in Soviet-controlled East Berlin. Brecht, one of our connections—a bridge between our dissimilar worlds.

"It took me months to find this particular record," Wolfdieter said.

I ripped open the thin East German gift-wrap, the texture of toilet paper. "'The Threepenny Opera!' I love it!"

"Maybe it's the last one in East Germany. With the original cast," he said.

We could not correspond openly, since letters might be censored. We could not communicate by telephone, as I did with my uncles and cousins in West Germany. It was this visit in person that brought us close again. And it had opened Stephanie's eyes as to how others lived in this world.

We continued in silence, on the long drive through darkened, empty streets. East Berlin was a ghost city with the scar of a hideous wall separating it from the West—dividing Berlin, dividing families, dividing brothers and sisters.

We arrived at No-Man's land. The wall was here obscured by barracks. The road was blocked by a barrier. When a car approached, it had to stop and submit to a thorough inspection. Then the heavy barrier would lift and allow the car to proceed. Towers flanked the road. We knew they were manned by armed soldiers. Anyone who tried to run the barrier would be shot. The soldiers shot to kill.

Wolfdieter stopped the car. This was as far as he could go. We got out, and I hugged the tall figure of my brother goodbye. All three of us got emotional.

Wolfdieter turned, and the two of us were left on the lone stretch where No-Man's Land begins. Wire loops swirled across the end of the long fenced-in walkway. The last view of my brother framed him encased in barbed wire. Klieg lights held him in a yellow circle. Heavy fog had risen and wrapped his body in a shroud.

"Mom, I'm afraid. This is really spooky." I held her hand a little tighter. My eyes were still on my brother, for a long time.

My brother, standing in the sulfurous light, fog sucking him into this surreal land, his figure a mere shadow now, in a trench coat, collar turned up against the cold, his hands buried in his pockets. I shook my head. No, this was not real, it was performance art; someone had put dry ice onto the stage, which sent up these swirls of mist. But reality intruded, I turned and waved. He took a hand out of his pocket and threw me a kiss, then he waved back.

This was real.

Stephanie walked closer to me. I held on to her as we continued between wire fences, then entered the building where we were to exchange our day pass for our American passports. The pungent smoke of Turkish cigarettes hung heavy beneath the low ceiling, making it hard to breathe. In line in front and behind us stood Turkish "guest-workers," returning from their Sunday fraternization with East German women. These women would "entertain" their foreign admirers on weekends in exchange for pantyhose and *real* coffee, chocolate bars, cigarettes.

A short guest worker behind me sidled up close. He breathed hot smoke onto my neck. I wheeled around, feeling the feathery brush of the tips of his mustache, and my stare threw angry darts into his clouded, heavy-lidded eyes. He backed off. When another Turk came up close to Stephanie, I stepped on his foot. He winced and lifted his foot massaging it through his Mid-Eastern loafer.

I clutched my brother's gift, and we walked to the table where everyone returning to the West had to open their bags for inspection.

The woman at the station nearest me was elderly, her short-cropped hair matched the gray of her uniform. Her heavy face, the color of stale white bread, showed no signs of ever having laughed.

"Guten Abend," I smiled a good evening at her.

The policewoman grunted. She eyed my hand. I twisted my wedding band to face my palm; its diamonds, though small, seemed ostentatious in this poor country. I need not have been concerned, her eye fastened on the record. With one quick move she snatched it from me. She tore through the rewrapped paper and ripped the flap open.

"Nein!" she shouted. "You can't take that with you. *Verboten!*"

"Give it back! Please! Don't take it from me—" I reached for the record. "My brother gave it to me!" My voice rose in pitch. "I love Bertolt Brecht. It's a recording of 'The Threepenny Opera' of the original production." As if she cared? I sniffed, blew my nose, and added, "With Lotte Lenya."

Stephanie stood by my side. She held onto my arm, and I knew she was even more scared now.

My eyes bored into the policewoman who returned my stare. Her expression was blank. I inhaled, straightened my back. I heard myself speak, every syllable a monotone staccato.

"I would like to keep this record. It will remind me of my brother and the love we share for Brecht. After all, he is your most famous Communist writer. I am sure that your government won't mind me taking Brecht's work out of Germany, to America."

"And your brother lives here?"

What had I done? Now I got frightened. *Would she ask for his name? His address?* Meekly I answered, "Yes. And we both love Bertolt Brecht."

I watched her facial muscles change. The jutting point of her chin softened and withdrew into the folds of flesh wrapping her neck. She handed the record back to me and gently put her hand on my shoulder.

"*Hier.* Take it! *Schnell!*" She indicated I should quickly hide it underneath my long jacket.

I could not believe my small victory. She was human, after all.

Clutching our American passports, and with my elbow squeezing the record to my waist while my free hand held on to Stephanie, we were on our way.

After a few more steps we reached Checkpoint Charlie, the lonely post, painted an innocent white. The tall black American MP glanced at our passports, flashed a big-toothed grin, and said, "Welcome to the land of the free." Then he noticed several of the Turks lurking around, observing us. The streets in this part of West Berlin were as deserted as the ones in East Berlin. We would have to walk several blocks to reach public transportation. "Hey, ladies. It's not safe for you at this hour. Wait just a minute, I'll call you a taxi." A minute later he returned from the building and gave us a thumbs up sign. Stephanie did the same, and again he grinned with his shiny whites, saying, "Taxi's on the way." I felt like falling around his neck and giving him a big thank-you smack on the cheek, but that would not have been appropriate.

When we climbed into the taxi, the Turks slunk off, the MP waved, and we waved back. Stephanie squeezed my hand, and I took a deep breath. Yes, it was the same fog-laden air, but here in the West it was easier to breathe.

When we were finally in bed, Stephanie whispered, "I can't believe how sweet these people are."

"Your uncle Wolfdieter and Babs?"

"Yes. They are so giving, and they don't have anything at all."

"They have a comfortable place. They treated us to a great meal."

"I don't mean that," she said. "They remind me of the lions in the Berlin Zoo, the two we saw yesterday. Remember? They have enough to eat and a comfy place to sleep, but they can't go anywhere. They're prisoners, when they really would like to be free and get back to Africa. They have such sad eyes." And then she added after a short pause, "The lions in the zoo."

After our visit to Berlin, Stephanie and I went to Usingen, a small town in the Taunus Mountains, some twenty miles or so north of Frankfurt am Main. Mother's eldest brother, my Uncle Richard, had died ten years ago, and I planned to have Stephanie meet Reverend Hans Ernst, a Lutheran pastor whom I had met at my uncle's funeral in 1972. We had carried on a lively correspondence over the past few years, and he was interested in meeting my daughter, in whose recovery process he had taken a special interest. It made sense we'd stop here on our way to the airport in Frankfurt. He had a doctorate in theology, and I found him to be a vastly learned man, able to interpret the Bible from its original texts—in Aramaic, in Hebrew, and in Greek. He was open to my many questions centered on the variant points of view of Christianity. But he mainly had given me hope as to Stephanie's future, based on his experience with a niece who had suffered brain damage many years ago from encephalitis caused by measles. The niece was now studying to be a nurse, and she was doing well.

"Stephanie will make it," he said. "It all takes time and patience."

He had grown up on a farm, and he took us to a farmhouse next door, where he showed Stephanie the neighbors' prized sow. He placed one of the piglets in her arms and let her feel its warmth and soft skin. Then he took us to the barn where cows were being milked, where the diverse scent of cows and milk, of fresh straw and dung was a new experience for Steff and for me. She asked if she could milk a cow—not easy with her partially paralyzed right hand. When she grabbed the cow's teats, the cow looked askance over her black-and-white bovine shoulder at Steffi, mooing with displeasure, and then slapped Stephanie's face with her dung-spattered tail.

"Ugh!" Stephanie cried out, jumping up. "Mom, where is there a bathroom? I have to wash up."

Later, Pastor Ernst walked with us through the woods and the fertile valley's wheat fields, sprouting green arrows of new growth. There were apple orchards now in a soft pink bloom, which later floated into my inner vision when Pastor Ernst served us the famous Frankfurter apple wine, grown only in this region. We were served the slender Frankfurter Würstchen and washed them down with the apple wine. Stephanie was served apple cider.

The reverend was a widower in his late sixties, but I felt as if I were in my own youth again, walking through forests with my father, who had given me my first lessons of nature observed. I felt sad that Pastor Ernst lived so far from us. He would have filled a vacancy in Stephanie's life, that of a kindly grandfather who could teach her lessons of simplicity, of country living, that her city-dwelling grandfather in Chattanooga could not provide. Pastor Ernst invited us to the rectory to have lunch after the church service, and Stephanie helped his housekeeper with the dishes, only using her left hand.

I thought of my complicated life with Marvin. Pastor Ernst saw the tears in my eyes and gently took my hand. I opened up to him and told him about my marital situation.

"Don't do anything rash," he counseled. "You've been married for twenty-one years, and Stephanie needs a father and a mother. I will pray for you that Marvin finds a way to break up with his cousin. I think you should show patience and forgiveness. Leaving him now would be premature."

I was grateful for his advice, which echoed my own intuitive feelings.

We flew to Rome next, where Stephanie's cousin Tracy was spending a semester studying art history, and flamboyant Aunt Farol was expected to arrive any day.

I reflected on our trip so far, and at that moment Stephanie appeared from the bathroom, her face flushed rosy from the shower, wearing one of the fluffy bathrobes the hotel provided. "Mom," she said, coming closer. "When I am traveling I don't feel handicapped. That is such a good feeling. Even Pastor Ernst's housekeeper didn't remark that I used only one hand drying the dishes. Well, I sort of held them in my right hand, but it was hard not to drop them. People never stare at my hand as they often do back home. And I feel I learn so much, it is great traveling with you."

"Oh, wow, that makes me so happy to hear you say that. I thought maybe I was selfish to drag you along on this trip. Did you understand, really understand the difference of living in East Berlin and West Berlin?"

She looked at me as if I were a bit daft. "But of course. They are in prison, and we are free, and West Berlin is free. It is not difficult to understand. And Mom, I will have lots of stories to tell when I get back. I am happy, really happy you took me along."

We stayed in the same hotel with Farol, but for the most part, Stephanie and I were on our own. It was Easter week, and many places and museums were closed, but we had fun walking through the streets where elegant boutiques were located near fabled landmarks. We went to the Trevi Fountain into which Stephanie threw exactly three coins, and the Coliseum where she wanted to pick up one of the many feral cats that roam the ruins. Maybe they were reincarnated ghosts of lions past. When I took her to the Sistine Chapel, she promptly flopped to the floor on her back to view the ceiling—making me laugh behind my hand. I did not have the heart to scold her, as I did her father, when he did the very same thing when we were in Rome on our honeymoon. A guard approached, ready to rebuke her, but Stephanie leapt to her feet, held her arms out wide, and smiled. She disarmed the guard, and he smiled back.

On Easter Sunday, we went to the Piazza San Pietro at the Vatican and stood with hundreds of thousands to hear Pope John Paul II deliver his Easter address. The pope appeared on his balcony. From our vantage point he was a small speck, much like a fly on a windowsill, while he addressed the crowd in many languages. I seem to recall it came close to thirty-two. The crowd jostled and I clung to my purse, while Stephanie held on to me. Then I had to rescue her from a young man who pinched her bottom, which effectively broke the sacred mood that had enveloped us as we received the words of the pope and his benediction.

In the evening, when Farol and I were alone for a while, she confessed that she had known about Marvin and Judith from the start, since she had been at the same family gathering where the two had begun their affair. She confessed she had meddled and was partially guilty for enabling the cousins to begin the affair. Now she was sorry. I knew she liked to stir things up, as if life was not crazy enough. I forgave her, since her sincerity seemed genuine. She was truly sorry for what she had started. She had earlier believed it would be a brief fling and regretted that she had done nothing to stop it. Farol now promised she would try and talk sense to her brother.

Soon our three weeks in Europe came to an end, and we returned home. Construction on the remodeling of our garden was in full swing, and the heaped dirt and broken concrete reminded me of my own torn and scrambled life.

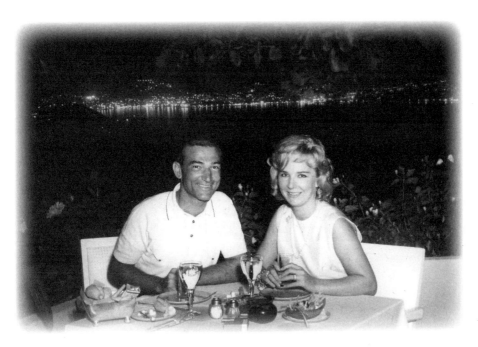

Marvin and Karin in early times in Acapulco, 1969

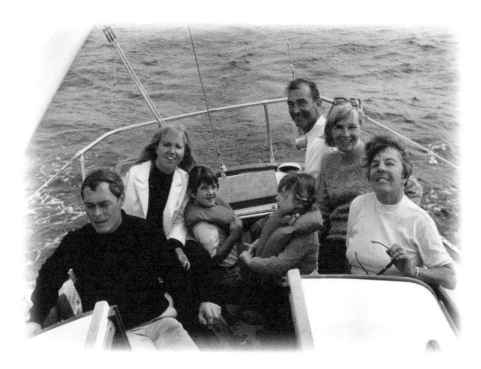

Marvin, Karin, Grandma Astrid, Steven, Stephanie, and
friends on a sailboat, 1970, photo by Heidrun Krings

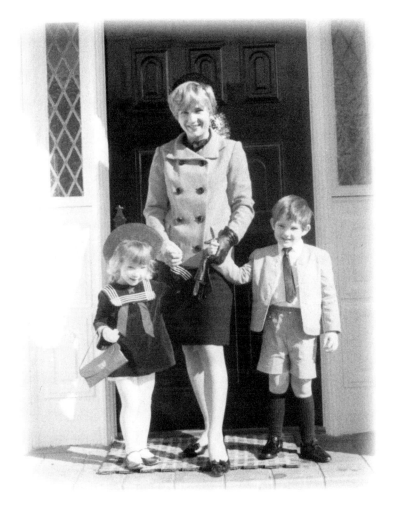

Karin, Stephanie, and Steven in front
of the house in Beverly Hills, 1967

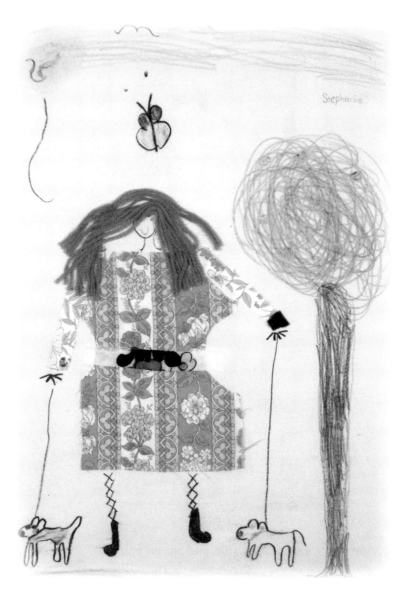

Stephanie's collage, made when she was six

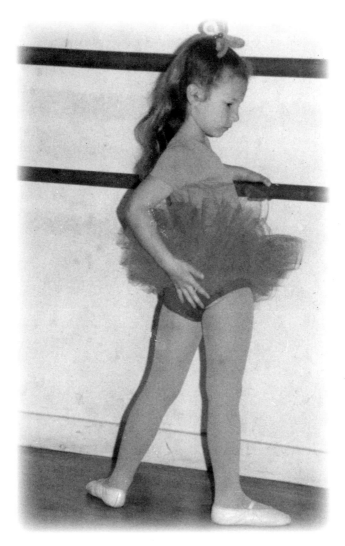

Stephanie in ballet class before her illness, 1969

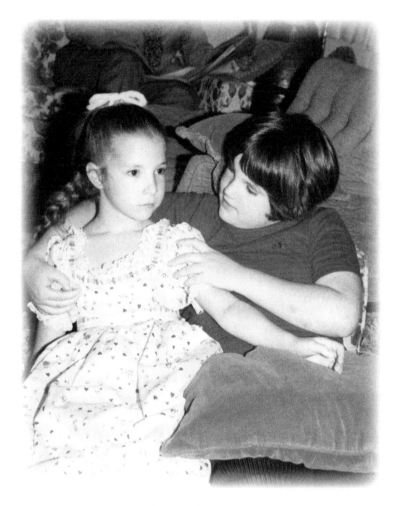

Stephanie after her coma

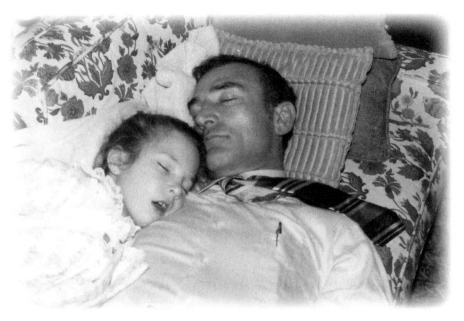

Stephanie and her dad napping in the afternoon
after she came home from the hospital, 1971

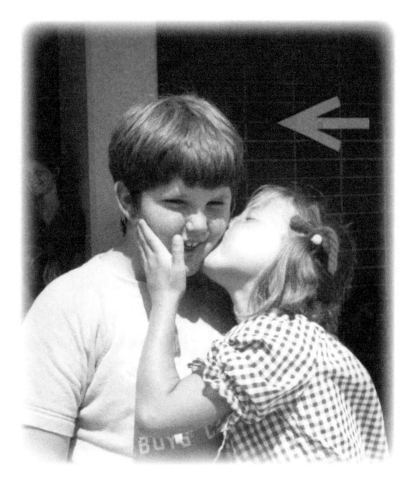

Stephanie kissing her brother, Steven, hello after
his homecoming from summer camp, 1972

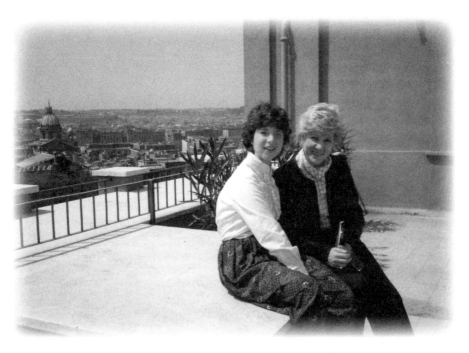

Stephanie and Aunt Farol in Rome, April 1982

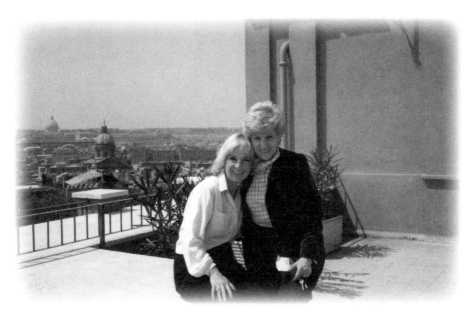

Farol and Karin on hotel terrace in Rome when Farol confessed
her role in getting Marvin and Judith together, April 1982

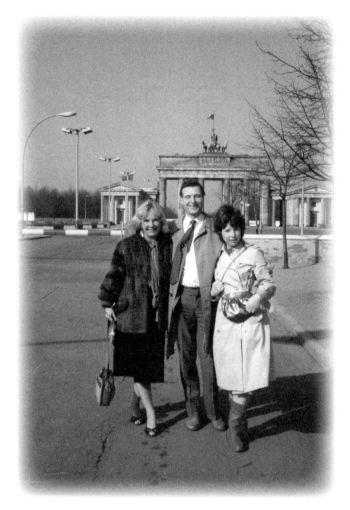

Karin, her brother Wolfdieter, and Stephanie
in East Berlin at Brandenburg Gate, 1982

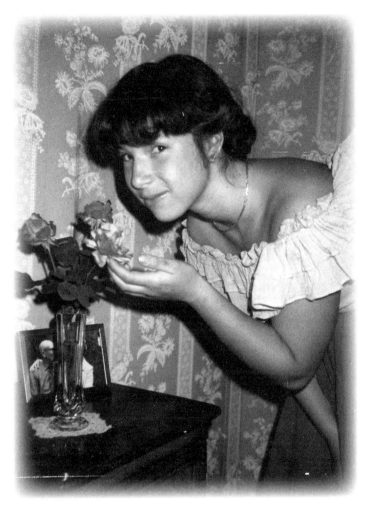

Stephanie in the old house in Beverly Hills, 1984

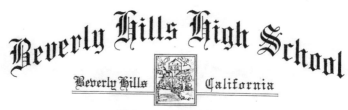

Beverly Hills High School

Beverly Hills · California

This certifies that

Stephanie Finell

has completed the course of study prescribed by the Board of Education of the Beverly Hills Unified School District and on the recommendation of the faculty is awarded this

Diploma

Given at Beverly Hills, California, this month of June, nineteen hundred eighty-three

Max Factor
President, Board of Education

Leon M. Lessinger
Superintendent of Schools

Sol Levine
Principal

Stephanie's high school certificate, 1983

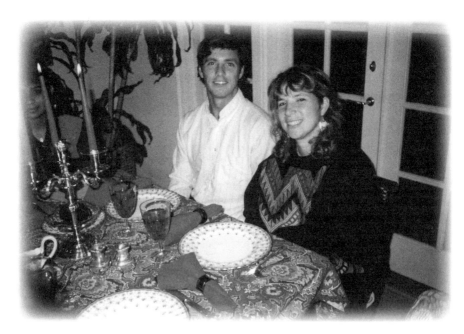

Stephanie and Loren, Christmas 1993

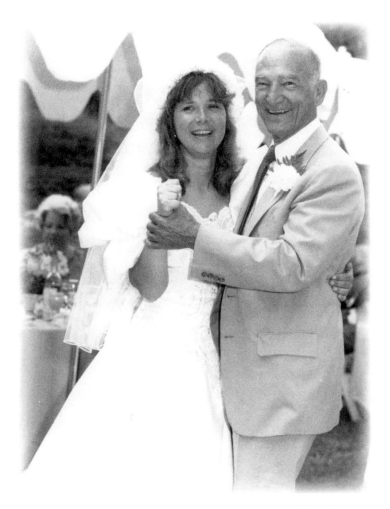

Stephanie dancing with her father on her wedding day,
May 1992. He was not wearing a tux as he'd promised.

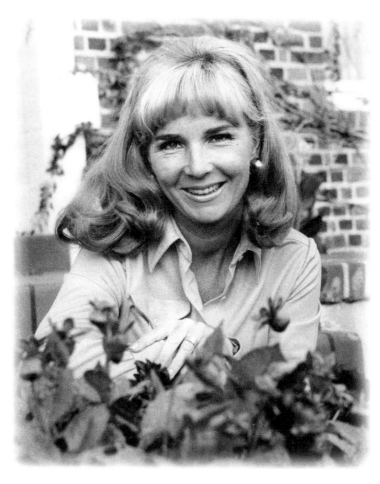

Karin at forty, photo by Heidrun Krings

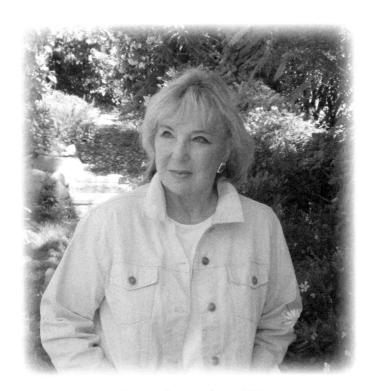

Karin in her garden, 2007

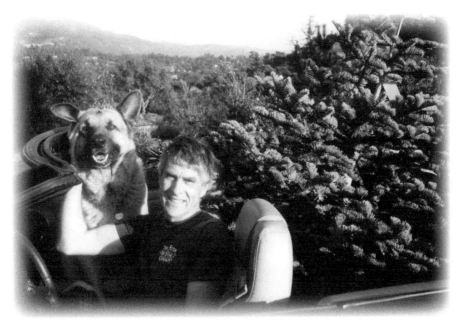

Martin and Aldo

Chapter Seventeen

No More Songs

After Stephanie and I returned from Europe, Marvin was loving and attentive and seemed to make an effort to repair our marriage. He did not tell me that he had broken up with Judith, but he was home most evenings, and we spent many a weekend in a condo on Lido Isle, an enclave of Newport Beach, about seventy miles south of Los Angeles. We still owned the condo in Century City, which Marvin said he had bought as an investment. When he told me he had leased this condo a few months ago, I wondered why he had signed a lease for two years, without discussing it with me. A few years ago he had started a business in Costa Mesa, and at that time we had rented Barry Goldwater's apartment in the Balboa Bay Club. Now there was no such reason. It puzzled me why he spent so much money.

On the first weekend on Lido Isle, Marvin surprised me with flower arrangements in the bedroom and the living room, and a small one in the bathroom. I was touched by his thoughtfulness. We bought plants for the condo, hung paintings, making it home.

Summer had come, and we spent fun-filled days there with Stephanie and her friends Michelle and Hugi. Steven visited us upon occasion. Friends and relatives from Europe stayed with us. I felt safe in this condo, knowing that Judith lived over an hour's travel north of us. No quickie escapes to her were possible.

We grew to love the condo by the bay, although there wasn't much of a beach, not more than a narrow band of sand leading to a slim arm of the canal surrounding the island on this side. From here we watched ducks and boats glide by. We liked the foggy mornings best. Then the condo filled with warmth and gemütlichkeit. Yes, coziness.

The fog metamorphosed boats into ghost ships. Ships' horns mourned, sailboats drifted unseen out to sea—known only by the sound of their stanchions clanking. Steffi and I jogged along the strip of sand and came back to a fire crackling in the fireplace, steaming java in the coffee maker, the Sunday paper spread over table and floor, with Marvin alternating between the sports pages and reading the funnies to Stephanie.

It was October now, and the remodeling of the front garden of our house was finished, but work was still going on in the lower level of the garden behind the house. A Jacuzzi and goldfish pond replete with waterfall were also new additions, now completed.

I had hoped we'd go to Lido Isle this weekend, but then Marvin had been gone for the last two days. He left without taking a suitcase and did not tell me where he was going. I worried. He was drinking heavily again, and I was afraid he might have blacked out somewhere. Or maybe he was at Judith's apartment? Friday afternoon came, and the contractor needed to be paid—there was no Marvin to pay him.

Stephanie might have suspected something was wrong, but she still did not know about Judith.

By Saturday morning she too began to worry. "Mom, where's Dad?"

"He's not at our condo in Newport, Steff. I called several times. No answer."

"I want to be with Dad," Stephanie sulked. "Maybe he'll. . .then. . ., can you and I go to our condo?"

"Well. . .sure, that's an idea. Get away for the weekend. Go then, get ready."

I left Marvin a note, in case he came home after we had left. As I packed a few things, doubts arose. I thought: Please, please, Powers that be, don't have him show up at the condo with *her*. I dismissed the fleeting thought. A while back he once had gone to Santa Barbara for two days without telling me in advance. Maybe he had the urge to go out of town and took Judith. The condo would be a good place for Stephanie and me to relax. Marvin was a man of good manners. He wouldn't take *her* to our family weekend-place. No, he would not. The condo was a perfect place.

Soon Stephanie and I were on our way. The silver car seemed to know its way, winding west on Sunset, then easing onto the San Diego Freeway, heading south. We sang "Michael Row the Boat Ashore—" and harmonized, and I told her stories. With Stephanie at my side, the drive became bearable. I hated the crowded Interstate 405, and the brown soupy air till we had passed through Long Beach and its oil refineries. Shortly after Costa Mesa the landscape opened, and we turned off for Newport Beach.

We traveled an endlessly wide boulevard past low-slung office buildings and stores, past gasoline stations and fast food places. Past the monotony of suburbia.

Then thoughts flashed through my head. I imagined Marvin and his cousin in the condo. With this, my heart went crazy, jumped a beat, raced. Bad habit,

Karin, this imagining of scenes. Had I not phoned several times? He won't be there. Am I really sure? What if he is there?

I looked at Stephanie. My child. I felt a wave of warmth rise in my body, which moments ago had felt cold and made me shiver. I reached for her hand and squeezed.

We passed a gun shop on the left side of the road, not far from our turnoff to Lido Isle. I swerved the car in a sudden left turn, swung into the parking area, came to a halt in front of the display window. I sat slumped in my seat, my nerves raw.

As if in a trance, I stared through the windshield. At guns. There were so many different kinds. My eyes fastened on a large one. It looked sensual. The black handle was shaped in an aesthetic curve, with the long silver metal jutting out ready to kill. But then I spotted a small second-hand revolver with a mother-of-pearl handle. It was almost beautiful, if one did not associate it with being an instrument of death.

All I had to do was—leave Stephanie in the car for a few minutes, go inside, buy the pretty little pearl-handled gun, buy some ammunition, have the salesman show me how to load the thing and, voilà, I'd be prepared.

Moments ago I had felt dead, frozen, now hatred made me burn. My insides felt like molten lava, viscous, vicious, consuming my reason. I was surprised to find myself capable of such passion, such uncontrollable lust for revenge. I closed my eyes, gritted my teeth. *Jesus, please help, I must get myself under control.*

Stephanie tugged at my arm. "Mom, why are we here?"

My eyes opened to the sight of guns.

Her question startled me. I did not tell her my thoughts.

And again she touched my sleeve. "Mom—?"

I shook my head, dispelling visions.

Why are we here?

Was I going to explain to her that Daddy, her beloved Daddy, had a mistress, Stephanie's own relative, his first cousin? Was I going to tell her, that if I found them in our condo, I would kill them both?

What was happening to me? How low had I sunk? I buried my head in my arms, shaking.

"What's wrong Mom? You're crying!" Her words were half accusation, half question, partially comforting.

Pull yourself together, Karin. I wiped my eyes with a Kleenex. Smudges of mascara clung to white. My nose clogged up. I sniffed. I heard myself laugh, sounding dry and sarcastic. My thoughts flew to Marvin and to "her." I felt the heat of hatred rise again. *If I find them, they'll be dead.* My smile broadened. Then it froze. I would wind up in the Sybil Brandt jail. What irony. I know Sybil Brandt! I had met her at the Wymans' house. I could not take care of Stephanie from jail. What would happen to my child?

She would be put into an institution.

An invisible bucket of ice water thrown by an invisible hand brought me back to reality. I turned the key in the ignition, the motor caught, purred. I slammed the gears into reverse, screeched into traffic, made a U-turn against all rules, and drove on to our condo.

Stephanie's earlier question remained unanswered as she looked at me askance.

"You sure act funny, Mom!"

She was right. I drove in less than five minutes from the gun shop and across the bridge to Lido Isle. I slid the card key into the slot, the heavy gates to the parking area swung open, the car screeched around a curve, and rolled into our assigned parking spot.

Thank you God, Marvin's car was nowhere in sight.

The key turned the lock of the apartment with ease. The door opened halfway, when the shadow of a woman came flying, Judith. She pressed against the door, trying to bar our entry. I put my foot in the entrance and swept her aside.

"You can't come in," she blasted in a sharp, yet at the same time, hushed voice. Adding with agitation, "No, you can't—" Then her voice trailed off as I pushed beyond her without a word. Stephanie seemed unsure but followed me, her eyes fastened to the carpet as though looking for something she had lost.

"He's drying out. He can't be upset. He'll start drinking again, you don't want to have his death on your hands, do you?" Judith screamed.

Stephanie's head swiveled from looking at this cousin to me.

"This is our apartment. I am here to see my husband," I said.

A few short steps took me to our bedroom. There was husband and father lying in our bed. The comforter I'd bought a couple of weeks ago was pulled up to his chin. The flower pattern wobbled like Jell-O when the bowl is moved, drawn as it was over Marvin's trembling body. He smiled—of all things. Clown-like. An apologetic smile. He looked unrecognizable. His face was flushed, swollen to the point of looking as though the skin would pop like that of a tomato held over a flame. He was wet with sweat, looking at me as if he were seeing a ghost. I remembered the frogs on my walk with Wolfdieter in Berlin. He reminded me of a large red frog. Again I thought, *How ironic, Marvin, he who had been my Prince Charming.*

My hatred had popped like a balloon. I felt detached and just a little sad for him, as if I were watching a movie.

"Hi, honey—," he said.

Honey, yes, that's what he called me.

Judy stood in the open doorway. Her hands were twisting the ankle-length blue denim skirt she wore. I noticed a smudge of mustard on the gray of her flower patterned cotton blouse. How strange that I would notice details like that at that time. Her feet were bare, small, bony feet, tipped by scarlet toenails.

"I insist. You must go," she said, stomping her right foot. "Now. This very moment."

I stared at her in silence. Not moving.

I turned to my husband, "Marvin, why didn't you answer the phone? You promised you would if you were in the condo. You could have spared Stephanie and me this—"

"I can't—I can't talk on the phone. I'm trying to get off the booze—God, it's so hard." He was near tears. Again I felt sorry for him. At the same time I felt angry with myself. I had no business feeling compassion for this man.

"Where's your car? We wouldn't have come in, had I seen it."

"I had a flat. It's in the gas station by the bridge."

I straightened up, trying to look taller and to sound authoritative. "You are coming home with me. Now! You can dry out at home."

"No, honey—" *Why does he keep calling me "honey"?* "I can't. Sorry, I really can't."

"He can't," chimed the echo, Judith. Her small frame advanced one hesitating step. "He has to be kept quiet. Can't be moved. If he doesn't make it now, he'll start drinking again. You know what that will mean. His liver is at the point of not regenerating. He'll die."

I looked at her, riddling her body with bullets, killing her with the imaginary gun I had not bought.

Looking frightened, Stephanie said, "Daddy, please, get well!"

"I'll come home day after tomorrow. Monday morning, early." The sweat made him look wet, yet his voice sounded dry, like brittle parchment. He looked at me, "I promise. Everything will be all right, honey." *Again that damn "honey"!* "I promise!"

"Yes, of course. I can believe your promise."

"I do, I promise."

Stephanie tugged at my sleeve and, pointing to her father, said she wanted to kiss him goodbye. I nodded.

"We'll go," I said. "I expect you Monday morning." I turned to Judy. "Give him plenty of tea with lots of honey (the irony of having to use *that* word) and some lemon. That's what he needs when he's drying out. I nursed him through this six months ago. If his body doesn't get the accustomed amount of alcohol, it must get its sugar in another form. And give him plenty of vitamins. Especially C."

"Yes, tell her," Marvin said, "She doesn't know."

Judy shot angry looks toward Marvin and me. Her eyes narrowed, her lips stretched into a clenched, thin line.

Marvin had remembered that earlier drying out period. He had been sent to Cedars for alcohol abuse by his doctor. Three hours later he was back home. It surprised me, he'd been scheduled to be at the hospital for at least ten days. He drew me to him, nuzzled my neck as he threw off his clothes, and climbed into bed. He said to me then, "I want to be home when I do this, with my favorite German nurse to take care of me. I have the will power. I can do it right here, in my own home."

It had not been easy. He had delirium, fever, sweats, horrible nightmares. I nursed him through three days of hell. Then suddenly he recovered and felt weakened, but normal. And he stayed off alcohol for nearly six months, but then, drinking bouts with Judith, each trying to match the other's consumption of Scotch, started his liver acting up again.

Stephanie now marched to the bed, kissed her father, then wiped off his sweat from her face with the back of her hand. Judy leaned against the door, hands planted at her waist, looking exasperated and disapproving. We walked out of the room. The front door fell shut behind us with a clang.

Stephanie kept crying on our drive back to Beverly Hills. She seemed instinctively to understand the situation, but she saw it all as if through veils. "Who is this Judith?" she asked. "What is she doing in our condo with Dad?"

I could not answer. I choked and shook my head. "Later, Stephanie, I'll tell you later," I managed to say.

I have often thought about that day. It was one of those times when you can choose one path or choose quite another, a crossroad. If I had thrown her out (if need be by calling the police, since it was *our* condo she was in), it might have saved our marriage. But I didn't want to fight for him. *He* had to be the strong one and fight for our marriage to survive.

Marvin did return that Monday, as he had promised. Another week passed when he announced, "I finally found a shrink who will treat her. When she's seen him a couple of times I will break up with her." The "she" of course was Judith. I smiled a disbelieving smile. He took me in his arms and stroked my hair. "We'll be all right, everything is going to be fine," he said.

Soon after Stephanie's birthday in November, she entered my study, her brown eyes watery. "Mom, is Dad mad at me or something? He won't talk to me. . .just kinda pushes me away."

"Maybe it's hard for him. . .not drinking anymore. He's quite a guy, to quit cold turkey like that."

"That's not it. I don't know. He's acting so strange—"

"Yes. . .he has a lot on his mind."

"I know. Judith. That's what." Stephanie sounded surly. "When do you think Dad is going to be like *my* Dad again?"

"I don't know, sweetie. But, surprise! He's planning to take us to England for Christmas. Merry Old England, won't that be fun? We'll stay in the country, in one of those traditional inns where they have a real English Christmas, like out of—"

"Like out of *A Christmas Carol*?"

"Exactly."

"Hm." She paused. "I don't want to go, Mom. Steven's baby is going to be born soon—that'll be so cute. A baby under the Christmas tree."

"Yes, it would be. But I think it's important we go to England with your father." I didn't tell her, but somehow I felt that Marvin had planned this trip to be far from the temptation of seeing *her* again during the holidays.

The tickets for the trip arrived, and soon Stephanie and I were busy shopping for proper clothes. We would be staying at the Lygon Arms, a seventeenth-century country inn in Broadway, in the Cotswolds.

We rented a car in London and drove through a wintry but surprisingly green countryside to the Lygon Arms. Helen Reddy's voice came over the radio, singing "You and me against the world—" while Stephanie sang along with the radio, then saying, "You too Mommy, you sing it too, remember, it's our song."

"Your song?" Marvin shouted and turned the radio off. Stephanie looked angry and surprised, and I sat as if dumb struck. Was he jealous that Stephanie and I had bonded more closely than ever during the last few months? I shook my head and let it pass. Let us keep the peace we seemed to have found and not evoke the ghost of Judith.

We arrived at the seventeenth-century and now modernized hotel, and it amazed us that Stephanie found her own room after the third time. We had shown her how to get there—traversing two corridors and one flight of stairs. Her room was in the new addition of the hotel, far from ours with the creaking and tilted seventeenth-century floor. Marvin remarked that she matured a little each time we took her from her accustomed surroundings.

"We must take her on more trips," he said.

None of the other guests seemed to have noticed her handicaps, well, perhaps when not using her fork and knife in the proper European manner of eating. But then, there were many Americans who cut their meat and then switched the knife from one hand to the other as she did. Other than that, she managed to hide the fact that her right hand was paralyzed, well. Stephanie charmed the English ladies with her good manners.

On Christmas Eve she wore a floor-length dress with a red-and-green tartan-plaid taffeta skirt. Its fitted bodice of dark-green velvet revealed lightly tanned shoulders, setting off the luster of a string of tiny pearls, a present from her grandparents. She wore her brown hair in loose ringlets, spiraling around her face. One of the older gentlemen called her a Pre-Raphaelite girl.

Christmas Eve

The dining room was decorated with holly and pine and red satin bows, the room was lit by wax candles, and the sumptuous six-course dinner with its varieties of wines put everyone in a holiday mood. Marvin had only half a glass of champagne to toast to Christmas. I admired him for not giving in to his urge to have a glass of Scotch, his favorite drink.

We decided to walk through the wintry night to attend the candlelight service at the parish church only a few blocks down the country road.

Marvin loved to sing, and his baritone sang harmony to my soprano's melody. Unfortunately my voice sounded a bit like sandpaper on wood, because vocal nodes had reappeared, now, for the second time in my life. Stephanie's sweet voice sang along with mine, making several of the parishioners smile at us, turning their heads. When we left the church, the male half of an older couple said, "When you sang, 'Silent Night,' your American voices rang out so splendidly."

A waxing moon lit the frosty night, and we decided to take a stroll through the narrow streets. As Stephanie quick-stepped ahead of us, two young village swains, emerging from a pub, grabbed her, whirled her around and sang "White Christmas," dreadfully off key. The taller one craned his muffler-draped neck and tried to kiss Stephanie. She pushed at him and ran off, he in pursuit, but we could see it was all in good-natured fun. Marvin and I caught up with them, while the second bloke kept repeating, "Sorry, sir, sorry, my mate here is a little bit blitzed tonight."

From then on, when someone acted tipsy, Stephanie mouthed, with a put-on British accent, "Oh, he's a little bit blitzed, you know!"

Soon a cloud seemed to lift from Marvin's spirit, and his smile became spontaneous and open. I hoped that, with each day, our marriage would grow stronger, and Marvin's memory of the dark-haired woman in Los Angeles would fade.

During our week's stay at the inn, we drove to Stratford-on-Avon on two occasions. We strolled through the streets with their half-timbered houses and bought several secondhand illustrated fairytale books for Stephanie in one of the quaint bookstores. In Stratford we saw a wonderful production of *The Tempest*. A few days later, we attended *King Lear*. These are two of my favorite plays. I did not have my Shakespeare plays with me, but before the theatre, I told her the story line of the plays as if they were fairytales. Stephanie learned to appreciate the language of Shakespeare, not by studying the bard in school, but by hearing the cadences and rhythm of his words as spoken on stage.

We drove to the castle ruins of Tintagel Head, built precariously on a narrow precipice of rock jutting into the turbulent Irish Sea. This castle on Cornwall's rugged coast reputedly is the birthplace of the legendary King Arthur, as well as the seat of Camelot, King Arthur's castle and the knights of his round table. In London we had seen the musical *Camelot*; and strolling amid the ruins, Stephanie and I let our imaginations drift to those days of yore, when knights in shining armor and fair ladies gowned in jewel-toned brocades strolled through these now roofless halls.

Suddenly I found myself alone. I stood on the narrow drawbridge, beneath me waves crashed against gray granite rocks. I called out for Stephanie, for Marvin, but the only answer reaching my ears was the hollow echo of my own voice bouncing back from the windswept, crumbling walls. I suddenly felt a surge of panic, of despair. I felt alone. Abandoned. *Had I already lost my husband? Maybe these recent days of happiness were an illusion?* Silly thoughts. He said he'd broken up with her, completely, and only last night when he held me in his arms, he whispered he loved me and how happy he was to be with me so completely again. Then why did I feel this intangible "something" between him and me? This dark-winged premonition? What if he were to change his mind again? I couldn't bear the thought of living without him. Wouldn't I do all concerned a favor by disappearing?

The sea foamed and roiled beneath the bridge, waves crashed onto the cliffs. I took off my wooly beret, my coat, folded everything in a neat bundle and put it on the bridge's wide rail. Finding my clothing would let Marvin know I had jumped from here. I took off my gloves and slid them underneath the coat. The north wind cut like a knife, I blew into my hands to keep them warm.

Just then Stephanie came running out of the castle gate, calling, "Mommy, Mom, where were you? We've been looking all over for you."

Marvin followed. "Where were you? We thought we lost you through a trap door or something." And then, looking at me, clad only in sweater and pants, he said, "Aren't you cold? You'd better put on your coat, woman, or you'll catch the death of pneumonia."

It was toward the end of January. We had been back for a couple of weeks, and I was not able to speak, other than with a rasp. By now the vocal nodes had grown very large and impaired my speech more than before. Dr. Feder, to whom I had confided my marital problems, believed the nodes were brought on by nervous tension tightening the vocal cords, and the constant friction caused the nodes to grow larger. He'd told me months ago that absolute voice rest was required for three weeks after the operation.

"Mrs. Finell," he had warned. "I will not remove the nodes until you reconcile with your husband, or if not, have separated for a while and adjusted to the new situation. You must know how important it is to remain tranquil during the recovery period."

He repeated the warning of the three weeks of utter quietness and tranquility, and like a teacher, he wagged his finger warning me, and Marvin too, who'd accompanied me to the scheduling appointment. I must not speak, not whisper, and not weep. Especially not weep, for then the vocal cords would tense up even more. He explained that there is a very fine lining on the vocal chords, and this is what produces the modality of sound. When scars form, the lining loses its elasticity and the sound produced would wobble. The voice would be hoarse. If I were to break any of his rules for voice rest, I would risk impairing my voice permanently.

Before the nodes developed, I had a nice singing voice. Marvin loved my singing at parties or when we were alone. My voice was not big, but I had a clear lyric soprano with a pleasant timbre. I studied voice as a teenager in Berlin on a scholarship, and I sang professionally for a short while. A month before emigrating to the United States I'd sung with a big band at a benefit concert for the German Olympics Committee in the Titania Palace, in Berlin, to an audience of over two thousand.

I loved to sing, and I did not want to lose my voice.

Dr. Feder performed the surgery in early February. He removed two oversized nodules from my vocal cords, and I lay recovering in Cedars-Sinai as many a man's dream—a silent woman. Flower arrangements brightened the room. I especially loved the spectacular array of roses in all conceivable shades of pink ranging to a deep red that Marvin and Stephanie signed, "With love, always—"

The second day after I came home from hospital, I asked Marvin—by writing on my yellow pad—to please take me to Smith's Market. The anesthetic still affected me, and I felt too weak and groggy to attempt shopping alone. My throat muscles hurt, and my entire body ached and felt leaden. I would rather have stayed in bed, but Marvin hated shopping and we were out of certain foods. We were driving down Whittier, had crossed Sunset, when I became aware of Marvin's irritable mood. I grabbed pad and pen and wrote, "You're acting so strange—?"

Silence.

Then, I opened Pandora's box, "Are you seeing Judith again?"

"Yes. Yes, I am," he said, forcing the steering wheel into making a screeching U-turn, heading back up Whittier for home. Then he added, "And I'm leaving you."

He dropped me off on the front steps. Then he drove off and out of sight.

Stephanie watched me stagger into the house. What she read on my face must have scared her. She took a step back, hesitated, then came up to me and wrapped her arms around me. I trembled, groped for Gloria, our housekeeper, and leaned on her as she helped me up the stairs. I kept shaking, as if I was in a fever. Gloria, who had been trained as a nurse in Guatemala, felt my pulse and shook her head. "I can not much feel it, Señora, so weak."

I shivered. I felt cold, down to my bones cold. This "from the inside-out cold" was frightening. I steered us to the bathroom. I needed a hot bath. Quick. Water soon filled the tub.

Gloria left, but Stephanie stayed. I was glad of it. I couldn't breathe, and I felt as if every ounce of life was ebbing from my body. Not at all like in Tintagel, when I had wanted to jump into the sea. Now, after Marvin had indeed left me, I wanted to live.

From one moment to the other, I knew that everything had changed. I had deluded myself. Marvin was no longer the man I married. He had become a stranger. I needed to live for Stephanie.

The water was scalding. I immersed myself up to my chin. Still, I felt frozen to my innermost being. When I lifted my arm, I noticed the tiny hairs on it standing upright among the goose bumps of my skin. Stephanie sat quietly at the edge of the tub. She caressed my hair, my face. I couldn't speak, couldn't let her know what was happening. She leaned her forehead against mine, and I knew she was aware of something wrong. Terribly wrong. Then she asked, "Mom, what happened? Is Dad gone?"

I nodded. Stephanie twisted her mouth into strange shapes. She chewed on her lips, then stretched them into a taut line. Her eyes closed. She made no sound, joining my silence. Finally she leaned over the tub and kissed my cheek, her honey brown hair mixing with my own, shoulder-length and blonde. She held her flushed face close to mine and continued running her fingers through my hair. The mirrored wall by the marble-enclosed tub showed two red-faced women, one young, one middle-aged, enveloped in steam, and two pairs of red-rimmed eyes, showing fear.

Being left by a husband after twenty-three years felt like a small death. I saw those years as a tall clay jar, and all the joys that once had filled it were emptied out and replaced in equal measure by pain.

Four weeks had passed since the operation, and I still could not speak beyond a rasp. It was as if the pain of loss kept knifing my throat, and fear of the future clogged it. My throat was not healing and I knew I would never be able to sing again.

But whom would I sing my love songs to now? To Stephanie?
Yes, but they would be songs of love, not love songs.

In April, two months after Marvin left me, I took Stephanie with me to visit Carmen and Alonso in Guadalajara. Carmen and I had been friends since before our respective marriages. I was her maid of honor at her wedding, and her eldest daughter's godmother. In Mexico I found solace, and Stephanie found a caring family who included her in their life. In Carmen's children, Stephanie found two brothers and two sisters. They called her their *gringa hermana*. We drank our fill of this atmosphere of understanding and love. After two weeks, we reluctantly returned to our large house, this once so warm and enfolding house that now felt cold and empty.

In June, Stephanie was to graduate from Clearview. She felt proud receiving a high school graduation certificate issued, not by but through Beverly Hills High School, which would have been her assigned school. The ceremony would take place at the Riviera Country Club. Stephanie bubbled over on the telephone to her father, telling him where and when. He called me back and told me to celebrate the event with a party.

"Will you be. . .bringing Judy?" I asked.

"No. We'll be visiting her daughter back in Connecticut at that time."

"You're not going to be here for Stephanie's graduation?"

"You know it's some Mickey Mouse kind of affair. That certificate doesn't mean anything."

" Mickey Mouse affair? Hey. . .just a minute." I felt myself get angrier by the minute. "It means a whole lot to Stephanie. That's what counts."

"Gotta go. You handle the invitations to the party. I'll pay for it. I bought her a very pretty necklace. That'll make her happy."

"A necklace! Paying for a party! Her daddy at her graduation would make her happy."

"Sorry, can't do it. Bye." Click. End of conversation.

At first Stephanie felt sad that her father would not be there to share her accomplishment, her joy. Then we began our preparations and mailed out invitations, and her anticipation overshadowed her sadness. The day arrived. When Stephanie received her certificate she was overcome with emotion. At the lectern she tripped over a step and reeled onto the podium. Mark, her age, a boy she'd had a crush on since both attended the Frostig Center, caught her. Then he offered her his arm. By now Stephanie's cap had slid partially off her head, covering her right eye rather rakishly. The blue graduation gown slid off her right shoulder, revealing the beige-lace dress underneath. All this on her right side, the side that was still partially paralyzed. She appeared as if she were slightly tipsy, and since I knew she was not, the sight was endearing.

Later, at the dinner in the Bel Air Bar and Grill, she acted composed and radiant and proud that she was now a "high school graduate."

She was nineteen, but she could not follow high school with college. I worried what the next step would be, now that her basic schooling had come to an end.

During the prior months Stephanie had helped me through my own pain and infused me with courage to build a new life. I was proud of her and of her indomitable spirit. She had grown, not only into a lithe, lovely young woman but also into someone who was resilient and strong to face whatever the world might hold in store for her.

Chapter Eighteen

Of Lion Trees and Elephants

In my dream
I saw all these animals coming
so beautiful
the moment of my dream
> —Stephanie Finell

July 1983

Two years earlier I had visited Kenya with Marvin. Africa had entered my bones, and now they ached to return. On impulse, I decided to run off to this faraway land while I still had a viable credit card—and take Stephanie with me. Run away from the big house with its memories, our house that had become a tomb. I told Stephanie I had to get away from our surroundings, and Africa was as far away from Beverly Hills as one could get. And Stephanie understood that I was not only speaking of geography.

Stephanie had pored over my photos from Kenya, and she loved to hear stories about lions and elephants, but as the date for our journey grew closer, she felt uncertain about traveling so far from home. She had heard that in Africa sleeping sickness occurred, a type of encephalitis. I let her know I had informed myself of the risk by calling the Centers for Disease Control in Atlanta. I was given a description of the fly, what the bites looked like, and what to do in case one of us was bitten. That particular fly, the tsetse fly, is akin to our horsefly, a much more visible insect than the tiny mosquito that transmitted the Venezuelan encephalitis.

I looked forward to our four-week tour of Tanzania, the Seychelles Islands, and Kenya, and since I felt familiar with the latter country, I arranged for an extension to visit more of Kenya on our own.

After our first day in Arusha, Tanzania, Stephanie wrote to her friend Michelle:

> Dear Michy, I thought I wasn't going to like it, but guess what: I love it all. All. I saw lions in trees, imagine, in trees! And elephants and zebras, one of them was trapped, to be eaten by the people who are so very hungry. Poor thing. . .

This was written after our first game run, where the lions rested in trees, in the Acacia Arabica. They looked like furry pets, lazing on thorny branched hammocks. Stephanie would have liked to touch them, scratch them behind their tufted ears. But, when they yawned, displaying huge pointed teeth and a ravenous pink-throated cavity, she happily left the lions in their lion-trees.

We met our first elephants. Stephanie pointed to a large bull, saying, "Mom, look, that one has five legs!" Our fellow passengers in the Land Rover chuckled.

Then we saw our first zebras. They closely surrounded one of their herd, which was caught in a poacher's snare. The wire hung loosely around its neck, but its leg was caught in such a way that the animal could not move. It was touching to witness the herd's loyalty, crowding around one of their own, trying to protect it.

"Is she afraid, Mom?" Most animals were *she* to Stephanie.

"I think so. Animals get scared when they feel something is wrong. And this is wrong."

"When the butcher kills cows, or little lambs—for us to eat, I mean—are they afraid? Do the animals know what's going to happen to them?"

"Perhaps they have a premonition," I said.

"Somebody said, when we eat meat, we eat the animal's fear. That's bad. Now I know what that means. I won't have any more hamburgers."

I laughed and tweaked her cheek. "I'll remind you of that when we're back in the land of the Golden Arches."

Later, our guide reported the zebra incident to the game warden. His response was a shrug. The zebra would have been killed and butchered by the time the ranger could do anything about it.

Stephanie was appalled. But again I tried to explain that these people seldom get a taste of meat, that they live on a protein-deficient diet, and that money for the zebra hide would buy necessities for a family. Stephanie cried for the zebra, and perhaps for the poverty of these people. I believe she understood the difficulty of trying to sustain a world in balance for both humankind, and wild animals, in the face of so much poverty.

Sitting on our balcony we beheld the vast plain of the Serengeti amid the Great Rift Valley, broken by a broad silver band, Lake Manyara. A wide arrow of pink stretched into the silver—flamingoes. Thousands of them. Pink, pink, pink, like apple blossoms gently whipped onto a pond. The sky had filled with graying clouds, purpled with evening light; then suddenly it was dark. Night fell quickly, here, at the equator.

Even at this hour, birds sang their varied songs. We had seen a Rufous-naped lark today. Is that what we heard now? Singing one of the songs of Africa, melodic and unforgettable.

Salaam. Peace. A deep serenity enveloped the land, a stillness that filled us with wonder. This was the feeling that made me love Africa. And now this same feeling of peace and wonder filled my daughter.

After dinner in our hotel, we went to the adjoining room to have a cup of coffee and listen to the live band, and here, Stephanie met an eighteen-year old Hindu Tanzanian. He asked her to dance. After a few numbers both returned to the table. He shook my hand and introduced himself.

"My name is Damish," he said. And continuing in his distinct East Indian accent he announced, "I am pure Hindu, pure Hindu! In our faahmily there has never been anyone who is not Hindu."

I watched his round brown eyes traveling across Stephanie, from head to toe and up again.

He furrowed his brows as if in concentration and continued, "But I, I am modern man. Yes, modern. Well educated. I would consider marrying with European woman." He pointed to Stephanie.

"I'm American," Stephanie said, waving him on to sit down.

"But you are of European descent."

"American," she insisted. "A real mix. Mother is German, and my father is Jewish."

"Jewish? Ah, that is a good religion. The people of the Book."

"But I'm Episcopalian."

"Episcopalian?" Damish seemingly tasted each syllable while speaking. "Church of England? Ah, veddy good! I went to school from Episcopalian. Taught me much, good people." He shifted his somewhat protruding eyes to me, saying, "You, you are my mother now. I would like to marry with your daughter. All can be arranged, Mother."

Mother? Yes, I heard correctly; he called me *mother*. "Not so fast Damish, you are very nice, but—"

"You soon will meet my veddy own faahmily."

"Hold it, now. Hold it right there," I said, shaking my head, while Stephanie held a napkin in front of her mouth. I could tell by her mischievous look and her bobbing shoulders that she was trying to stifle a fit of laughter.

"Damish, in our country young men and women marry after they fall in love. They take time to get to know one another."

"I *am* in love!" By God, now he pounded his chest. "I am very much in love. I want to marry with your beautiful daughter because I cannot live without her."

Now Stephanie laughed openly. "Come on!" She gently pushed his ribs. "You've seen too many movies. I've danced with you twice!"

"But I know what I want."

"You're being silly." She waved her hand dismissing his remark. "Anyway, I don't know what I want." Stephanie rose from her chair, "Perhaps dance this number?" And with that she dragged him off to the dance floor.

I sat on the small banquette, back pressed against the wall and watched. A proper chaperon. I was impressed by how she handled him. For a while I listened to the orchestra (all were unschooled musicians), its beat, its sound. They improvised, made up melodies, took tribal songs, and elaborated upon a single melody with the syncopation of drums. I reveled in the music, and in watching Stephanie and Damish move with grace. Soon it was time to drag her off to our room (she could have danced all night), convincing her that we had to get up very early in the morning for another sight-seeing tour. We never met his parents or saw him again.

A month or so after we had returned to Los Angeles, an insured package arrived, which required Stephanie's signature. She felt very important and could not wait to tear open the brown paper with its fancy colorful stamps. A letter with a formal proposal was enclosed. And a small brown jewelry box appeared. When she opened it, a diamond ring sparkled. Jubilantly she put it on her finger, it fit! I was less then pleased, and I told her if it had any value, we would have to return it. She hid her left hand so I would not see the ring.

The next day we went to a jeweler friend, who smiled and said, "Yes, it is a fine, clear, one-carat Diamond. This guy in Tanzania is serious. What are you going to do"? Stephanie was with me and grabbed for the ring to put it back on her finger. "It's for me, I want to keep it."

"That is dishonest, Stephanie. Damish sent the ring hoping you will keep it and marry him. We have to send the ring back."

It took a while to make her understand. This little flirtation cost me a good penny in postage and insurance to return the ring, with a sweet, "Miss Stephanie regrets—" note, to extinguish once and for all the flame for Stephanie in this "pure Hindu" boy.

A few days after our arrival, in one of the tribal villages we visited, Stephanie met a young Maasai warrior, the village chief's firstborn. He wanted to buy her as his Number One wife. Steff answered, "Number One and only wife," believing like me, that this banter was in jest. After all, the young man spoke a fluent, if bookish English. Would he not be familiar with our customs? He repeated, "Number One." He then offered me thirty-five cows (which I later heard is an enormous amount), with bargaining as to the Tanzanian shilling and goats to follow.

Having read how much a Maasai chief had offered for Shirley McLaine, I asked for seventy-five cows. He looked Stephanie over, moved next to her, and seemed to measure her height against his own considerably tall frame.

"Yes. You are taller than I thought. I can offer a few more cows."

Stephanie laughed. "What? A woman is worth more cows when she's taller?"

He nodded. "Yes. That's our custom."

Stephanie walked away, shaking her head. He now agreed to pay fifty cows, when I caught a disapproving glance from our tour leader. He whispered that the taller a girl, the higher the bridal price—and, he is serious.

For the young Maasai this was *not* a game. How could I have been so insensitive? I quickly rescued the situation by telling the chief's son a little white lie. We would return in the company of Stephanie's father within two months; after all, her father should have the final say. The warrior nodded. He understood. *Her father.* A shadow fell over my mood. The words brought back our reality: her father no longer lived with us. Upon our return, we would be on our own.

Driving back to our lodge that evening, we experienced the Serengeti as a rolling ocean of golden grass upon which a playful god had placed granite islands looking like medieval castle ruins. Vegetation sprouted between rock crevices. Here water got trapped in hollows, and we watched from fairly close when a cheetah flashed its pink tongue to drink, darting watchful looks from its startling green eyes.

In the afternoon heat, the land itself appeared liquid, like a shimmering sea of vastness. At sunset, the grasslands burst into a fiery yellow and orange light, stenciling the umbrella trees like black paper cutouts onto the setting sun. Later, our seats on the verandah overlooked this panorama, and we watched as evening changed the colors from green to blue. We felt the land hold its breath in that brief moment when day becomes night, here, on the equator.

"Mom, I feel as if I belong here, it's so peaceful. I don't feel pressured to do this right, and that right. I want to stay here." I could not answer her but held her hand, and my breathing fell into rhythm with hers. Slow, regular, in harmony.

But not all was peace and quiet. Two days later, in the Ngorongoro Crater, two lionesses killed a wildebeest at the very moment our jeep reached the animals.

Our driver had spotted the herd of wildebeest race off in a cloud of dust. He floored the gas pedal and ripped over the savanna, knowing there would be lions, knowing there'd be a kill. He stopped. We were so close to the animals we could discern the lioness's eyelashes.

It all happened so fast. Within seconds. One lioness held down the head of the kicking and bellowing wildebeest, while the second one bit into the genitals, then ripped out the intestines. The first lioness, baring her teeth, began eating the animal's lips, then the tongue, in a bizarre kiss of death.

I tried to cover Stephanie's eyes with my hand, but she slapped it away and sat fascinated by the horror, staring with widened eyes. We would never forget the sounds of smacking, the snapping of sinews, ripping of fur, of skin, the cracking of bones. We would never forget the stench of the wildebeest's fear, the acrid urine, the metallic smell of blood.

Stephanie watched the struggle of life and death. The natural culling of a herd. This was not a movie. This was a lesson she could not have learned in biology class.

A few minutes later, our jeep got nearly rammed by the charge of a black rhino guarding her calf. She was annoyed by our driver who circled her and her offspring, and she charged us head-on. Stephanie sat next to the driver. The rhino came toward us at a gallop. I watched, paralyzed. The rhino's head grew large, larger. . .and then. . .? the driver made a strange "click" sound with his tongue. It sounded like a gunshot. The rhino stopped—straight on—a few feet from the jeep. Incredible. How could such a huge animal come to such an abrupt halt on a run like that? She threateningly lowered her head a few more times and watched us move on and out of her territory.

"Did you take a photo, Mom?" Stephanie asked, breathless, her eyes bright with excitement.

"Sorry, my hands were shaking. I was too scared."

"Yeah, wow, me too. But wasn't it great?"

There were times when Stephanie confused me. A few days ago, she loved Africa for the quiet, the harmony it exuded, and now she was attracted by the opposite, the cruelty of nature. I asked her, "Do you like this killing of one wildebeest by two lions? Isn't it a gruesome sight?

"No, Mom. You said yourself it is 'the natural culling of the herd.' The lions have to eat, and you said they eat the weakest of the animals. Isn't that nature? I hate it when I see a zebra trapped by the people, but then, they too are hungry and what are they to do?"

"Yes, that is a great problem in our world. Not enough food, too many people—"

An hour later the Land Rover climbed the two thousand feet to the rim of the Ngorongoro Crater. From this elevation of seventy-five hundred feet, we looked down as through a graying veil. Below us the valley and its Noah's Ark of animals lay shrouded in fog. The shadow of an Euphorbia Tree reached out with bony ghost fingers—its candlestick branches. A few Maasai walked the road, draped in orange to rust-colored *kangas*. I saw tears forming in Stephanie's eyes and asked, "What's wrong?"

"It's wonderful here, and tomorrow we have to leave."

"But we're going to the Seychelles, and then to Kenya." I tried to sound cheerful, but I too felt sad that our trip to Tanzania and its friendly people was coming to an end.

Mahé, the Seychelles

Stephanie was writing, pushing the yellow pad toward me.

"You've finished your letter to Dad already?"

"Yep. I write fast. Someday, I'm going to be a writer, just like you, Mom."

She handed me the letter. I was amazed how well Stephanie expressed herself. Her writing had certainly progressed in these last few months. Though her spelling and punctuation left much to be desired, her paper words sounded like those coming from her mouth. The legibility depended on her energy level. Today I found little to correct.

> Dear Dad,
>
> I love each and every day in Africa. Tanzania was incredibly beautiful. I feel so lucky to be here. We saw two lions kill a wildebeest; they say to see a lion kill is very rare. Well, your daughter, Stephanie Diane, saw one on her third day! And a rhino attacked our jeep. It was so exciting. My Walkman got stolen, but I don't mind, the people in Tanzania have nothing. They are so poor, you can't believe it. They trapped a zebra, to eat it. Part of all this is awful, but then, I'm learning a lot. A Hindu boy wanted to marry me. "I am pure Hindu," he said. I said, "Well, I'm pure American." And I told him, I'm half-Jewish, half-German, and Episcopalian, and guess what? He found everything to be just honky-dory. I just laughed.
>
> I miss you Dad, but am glad I am here and going to Kenya after this. Love and kisses, your daughter, Stephanie Diane.

I reflected on our trip, and how while traveling, Stephanie seemed to progress in many ways. In Tanzania something had opened in her, and I hoped it would not close off after we were back in the States, where she often felt so insecure.

Chapter Nineteen

The Heartbeat of the Earth

The plane winged us over the Indian Ocean back to Africa, to Kenya. We arrived at the

Ark, one of the game lodges high in the mountains, on July 30, Marvin's birthday.

"May I call Dad? Wish him a Happy Birthday?"

"There are no phones here, Pumpkin. Do you miss him?"

"Kinda."

I could see her eyes misting, and I knew she missed him. A lot. She tried to be brave. She had been her father's special little girl, dependent on his daily dose of attention and love. Even now, at nineteen, she was in some ways still a little girl who needed her daddy for hugs, for kisses, for guidance. What will happen when we return? Will she see more of him than during the previous few months? Will there be room for her in his new life with Judy? Will he take her to the places the three of us had frequented, the Dorothy Chandler Pavilion for a ballet or a concert? Would he take her along on weekends to La Costa where there was horseback riding and dancing? How would I react to such an arrangement? Would I feel jealous of "her" if Stephanie came back with enthusiastic praise, as she often did when people were kind to her? Questions, questions. I resolved to be accepting about the situation, and have Stephanie spend as much time with her father and Judy as they would want. I knew it was important for Stephanie's future relationships with men to feel close to her father and to respect him. I felt abandoned by my father and longed for him my entire life. I resolved this must not happen to Stephanie, if at all possible. At the same time I must discourage her from believing her father would come back. But she kept dreaming and wrote:

I hope, I hope,
That soon my Dad will wake up,
I hope, I hope,
And come back one day.

I turned my thoughts off. After all, we were still in Africa, far from our uncertainties. For now the peace of Africa had entered our being, and we felt in harmony. I thought of the earlier time when I was here with Marvin. I did not have the same connection to the spirit of things then. It was Stephanie who helped open my eyes and my heart.

At the Ark, at an altitude of nine thousand feet in the highlands of Kenya, it was cold. There was a slight drizzle at dusk while the animals trudged to the water hole. It was so quiet we dared not speak.

Suddenly Stephanie shouted, "I love you, Africa!" At the same time a bell sounded, signifying a large animal had arrived at the salt lick. We tapped our way in the semidarkness to the viewing terrace and stared at a huge leopard, green eyes flashing in the artificial light near the salt lick, his head bent low, eyes ever watchful, darting around his surroundings.

A black Servil cat sat on the railing, watching us, and as Stephanie reached out to pet it, the wild animal hissed. Steff jumped back, and the cat disappeared into the night.

We spent two more weeks visiting the Maasai Mara and several other national parks and then arrived back in Nairobi. From there we began traveling on our own. Our first destination was Mrs. Mitchell's tea plantation in Limuru.

The plantation lay at an elevation of seventy-two hundred feet, where the climate was ideal for growing tea in the tropics. Here Stephanie learned about colonial history from a Grand Old Lady, the daughter of one of Kenya's early British settlers.

Our taxi entered through high and massive wooden gates, looking as though they would lead us into a fortified Anglo-Saxon castle. The gates were heavily reinforced with thick, wide steel bands. A young Kikuyu gardener swung them open, and as we drove up, I marveled again at the impressive stone house, cozy looking despite its size, and with its green shutters seemingly more at home in the Cotswolds than here in Africa. Six sprinting, barking German shepherds chased our taxi (here they are called Alsatians), as well as several Rottweilers, another fierce German breed of herding dog now trained as guard dogs. The barking announced our arrival, the door to the house opened, and Mrs. Mitchell, who remembered me from my prior visit two years earlier, greeted us with open arms. The dogs now seemed to smile at us as well, and Stephanie, who loved dogs, ran toward them and began petting the most ferocious-looking Rottweiler. Moments earlier, the Kikuyu taxi driver had cautiously left the cab to open the doors for us, but surrounded by the dogs, who growled at him with their hackles raised, he practically flung our luggage out, quickly jumped back into his taxi, closed the doors, and left.

While a houseman took our luggage to our room, Mrs. Mitchell said, "You can stretch your legs before lunch," and invited us to follow her on a stroll through her prized garden. And a wonder of an English garden it was. We for-

got we were in Kenya as we admired the many European flowers and blooming shrubs. A riotous palette of blue, purple, and red hydrangeas vied for space
with carnations, lilies, sweet peas, and gladioli. When we arrived at Mrs. Mitchell's award-winning rose garden, the colors ranged from pure white to brilliant
yellow, from pink to deep violet, to almost black, then the orange-red of St.
Joseph's coat led to a spectacular intense variety, the color of a matador's cape.

The ringing of a bell told us it was time to return to the house, wash up, and
take our places at the large mahogany table for lunch. After the meal and a nap,
we walked through a primeval forest with our hostess, while a group of Colo-
bus monkeys—flashes of white and black fur—leapt from branch to branch
above us. Stephanie linked arms with Mrs. Mitchell as we marched below
the monkeys and listened to their mirth and Mrs. Mitchell's tales. She drew
a word portrait for us of her own beautiful mother, who had arrived by boat
in 1908.

"Father married her straight away, before she could change her mind."

"Why would she change her mind?"

"Oh. . .well, Stephanie, she was quite a proper lady. And here," Mrs. Mitchell's
arm swept wide, "where my father had his shack, there was nothing. Nothing.
All this came much later, with hard work."

"But if she came all this way, and she loved him, why wouldn't she have been
happy to stay?"

Mrs. Mitchell's laugh sounded somewhat uncertain. "She did stay. As for
love, she hardly knew him. That too came later, I suspect."

All this amazed Stephanie, and when we were alone, she mimicked the
British accent, swept her arm, and said, "Oh love, love comes later, much later,
I suspect."

The setting here was quite unreal, and not being former British colonials, we
felt misplaced. At dinnertime we met Mr. Mitchell, who had been the chief of
police in Nairobi before Kenya's independence. He was a big man, cordial and
dressed in a white dinner jacket. Dinner was eaten by candlelight, served by
a Kikuyu houseman wearing white gloves and carrying a heavy sterling silver
serving tray.

We had changed from pants into dresses for the semi-formal dinner. Stephanie looked sweet and old-fashioned in the soft glow of candlelight, wearing a
flowery voile dress baring her shoulders, as if she had stepped out of *Heat and
Dust*, a Merchant-Ivory film.

Africa became Stephanie's textbook. The Mitchells had told her about Uhuru, the fight for Kenyan independence. On December 12, 1963, Britain granted
Kenya self-rule. Steffi giggled, telling the Mitchells that she was born November 10 that year, so she was older than Kenya! Mrs. Mitchell laughed, but then
her face turned sad. Autonomy was a fact these former colonials had to live
with, a fact to be endured. The Mitchells had lost much of their plantation and
still, after all these years, had to live in fear of perhaps another uprising.

But years ago, Mrs. Mitchell's life was like pages taken out of Isaak Dinesen's autobiography, *Out of Africa*. She had attended many a party with Baroness Karen von Blixen (aka Isaak Dinesen) and told us anecdotes of her. She was an aristocrat and a rebel, just as she appears in her book. I had read certain passages from that book to Stephanie, which begins with the wonderful cadence: "I had a farm in Africa." Now Isaak Dinesen's pages sprang to life for both of us.

And the Leakys used to live next door to Mrs. Mitchell's parents. The anthropologist, Dr. Louis Leaky—who had here in Kenya discovered First Man—and she had played together as children.

Later, in bed, Stephanie said, "Mom, I would love to live here in Kenya." Then she thought for a while and said, "But then, it would be hard."

"Why?"

"Because, we'd probably have to live behind a big stone wall, like the Mitchells. Separated from the *real* people of Kenya. We wouldn't truly be part of it, I mean, of the whole of it."

"Yes, sad, but you are right," I said, kissing her good night.

As I closed my eyes, I thought how rapidly Stephanie was maturing on this trip—how she instinctively understood the undercurrents of a situation. Schoolwise she lacked education, but with her eyes and her heart she absorbed more education than many a high school graduate from an average California school.

After four days at the Mitchells' home, we rented a small hatchback Mazda and hired Joseph, a local Kikuyu driver. He was to drive us to Samburu and later to Lewa Downs, a forty-thousand-acre farm, now operating part-time as a tourist destination. This stay, too, I had arranged by telephone earlier. Marvin and I had been here two years ago.

We drove over carmine roads. Their dust left a coat of red on our car. Joseph pointed out the lush green fields of coffee growing in rich, volcanic soil. Stephanie asked, "Is that lady's, Isaac. . .something, coffee plantation near here? You know, the one who wrote about Africa.?"

How had she remembered that? If she had read it on a page, she would have forgotten it by today—no, an hour later. She remembered it because of Mrs. Mitchell's tales.

Joseph shook his head in a *No*. He either didn't know who the author was or didn't know where the farm had been located.

Then a splash of bright yellow fields burst into view, and wild oats wavered like silvery-blond hair, backlit by the sun. Acacia trees bore what appeared to be round fruit, but in fact these were weaver-bird nests, and we watched as the small birds flew in and out. Below the trees, arrogant-looking secretary birds stalked, mimicking officious government employees.

Near Samburu Lodge, we were suddenly confronted by a large herd of elephants, perhaps thirty, trumpeting, swinging their trunks, and heading our way. They soon caught up to us, and our hatchback seemed very small indeed. I remembered the story we had heard in Tanzania of what happened there about a month before our visit. An official from the Wildlife Federation was found trampled into a pile of unrecognizable tissue inside his flattened, compact rental car. Near the wreck lay a dead baby elephant. Those who found him speculated that he had driven too fast around a curve on the rough dirt road and inadvertently hit the little elephant. The mother elephant took her revenge. The car was the enemy, and she smashed it into a flat piece of metal, leaving the driver a mass of pulp.

Now elephants trudged past us on both sides, appearing much larger and more frightening than when seen from a safari jeep. They crowded protectively around the young in their group, watchfully turning their heads, small eyes moving within folds of skin focusing on us with suspicion. We were driving in sand now and the driver said we had to keep moving or we might get stuck. Stephanie grabbed my arm, squeezing hard. Was it fear? or the raw emotion of observing these wondrous animals at such a close range? The rough beauty of these huge pachyderms made us stare misty eyed.

Stephanie said, "The Maasai think that elephants have a soul like humans."

I looked at her, "You remembered what the tour guide told us?"

"Yes, because I think the Maasai are right. It is so beautiful to think that elephants are so caring."

I thought of what we had been told in Tanzania, that the Maasai thought elephants were the only animals that had a soul like a human. Living in close proximity with elephants, they had observed their social behavior. The members of one clan or group of elephants watched out for each other and guarded each other's young. Elephants even seemed to remember the death of a close relative, perhaps a mother, and when passing the place where the dead lay, would tenderly touch the bones of that dead family member with their trunks, even if the death had occurred several years earlier, seemingly grieving like we humans would.

Our little car kept moving slowly within the forest of huge trunks and elephant legs. The animals appeared to walk ponderously slow, but still they propelled themselves forward faster in the sand than our little car traveled. I was caught in a web of wonder. These animals possessed their own magical dichotomy, inspiring reverence while simultaneously, because of their sheer size, arousing fear.

And on they lumbered, leaving us in their giant shadows.

And on we drove, to Lewa Downs, this forty-thousand-acre farm composed mainly of savanna. David and Delia Craig were the owners. David had remained on the farm during the freedom uprising of Uhuru, which had been especially bloody here in the remote Northern Frontier District (the NFD) in Kenya, while Delia traveled to Britain with their children until it was safe for them to return.

David, remembering me from my earlier visit with Marvin, greeted us with outstretched arms. He held Stephanie's hand a little longer than he held mine, his eyes fixed upon the bangles she wore, woven of copper, brass and lead. "Our telephone is dead again. The damn lines are down," he said, touching one of her bangles. "My guess is, you're wearing them."

"We bought these on our way here, at the outdoor market in Isiolo," I explained.

"That's right. That's where the bastards sell them after they take the lines down. That's what they're made of, *my* telephone wires."

I watched Stephanie take her bracelets off. "You want them back?" she asked, offering them on her palm.

"For heaven's sake, what good would that do?"

"You're so upset about them."

David's grin spread as wide as his broad red face. From deep within his belly, he summoned up a laugh, shaking his tall square frame. Pointing at Stephanie, he declared between guffaws, "She's all right, your daughter. Yeah, sure, let's straighten out those wires and string them up again, eh?"

We went to register, wrote our names in the logbook, and were shown to our tent. Stephanie objected to the small shower tent located behind the larger sleeping tent. Yes, it was a little more primitive than I remembered, but I convinced her that a shower from a bucket with holes, hoisted up by one of the Samburu workmen, was preferable to reeking of perspiration.

A little while later we were back at the public area, and Stephanie saw the Craigs' giant baobab tree. She grabbed my arm to stop and pointed to the weird bulbous outcroppings from its trunk and the twisted and bizarre branches it extended like arms and grasping fingers.

She said, "Mom, this looks like the pictures in my fairytale book. The one you got me in England, doesn't it?"

She was referring to *Undine*, illustrated by Arthur Rackham, which we bought for her in Stratford on Avon in a little bookshop. All three of us were still together then, on our last Christmas trip before the divorce. My head spun. So much had happened since that happy time. Tears ran down my face, and I quickly wiped them with a tissue. "Mom, what did I say to make you cry? Don't cry. Please."

I tousled her hair. "You didn't say anything, sweetie. Well, it reminded me of the trip to the Lygam Arms and how happy we still were. As a family, with Dad."

"We're happy now, just you and I, aren't we?"

She put both arms around me and cradled her head on my shoulder. I felt like laughing and crying and hugged her close but noticed others close by and straightened up. "Yes we are. I've had so many happy hours with you on this trip. And Steffi, I'm amazed you remembered the *Undine* book. You always manage to surprise me."

We both kept looking at the "Rackham" tree, this baobab, half fauna and half flora, where the human-looking part was still in an enchanted state. As now outlined against the purple sky, the tree's knobby, enormous limbs looked spooky in the twilight.

Here Stephanie met Vanessa, a young blonde about Stephanie's age, who worked on the farm helping with tourists. She had arrived from England about one week earlier. Stephanie, upon hearing this, couldn't restrain herself from besting her. "I've been in Africa longer than you have."

When Vanessa asked which college Stephanie attended, Steff told her about her illness. The sadness of lost potential made me choke. The brain injury again cast its shadow.

I reminded myself that Stephanie's thoughts and words—but for occasional regressions into a childish rivalry, as with Vanessa—could express the secrets of the heart better than her father or I could. She was endowed with a perceptive insight into the core of things, to see their simplicity and beauty. She remembered the Rackham illustrations in her fairytale book, which proved she was still progressing. It seemed strange, however, that I mainly noticed these improvements when we were far from home.

It was still early. We awoke to the sound of neighing and hoofbeats. Someone, we guessed Kilai, a Maasai tracker and keeper of the horses, shouted a guttural command. Then we heard hooves galloping off.

The time had come to leave the comfort of the warm bed. The hot water bottle—just hours earlier a welcome friend—had become a clammy, cold, rubbery thing to be banished to the foot of the cot. A rustling of footsteps promised hot water steaming in two basins, inside the zip-down and zip-up wash tent.

The African day began with a frosty coolness at this altitude of fifty-two hundred feet, and dry air. It did not permit leisure while dressing. We leaped from the cot's cocoon, ran to the washroom, made a quick attempt at cleanliness, then back, zip-zip into the tent and into jeans, T-shirt, and sweater.

On our way to the mess tent, Stephanie suddenly grabbed my arm and bid us both stand still. She closed her eyes, and we breathed deeply, tasting the freshness of the morning tinged in orange light. Then we walked on, past thorn bushes and through savanna grass, spotting impalas and gazelles in the distance. Stephanie pointed to Mt. Kenya's peak, jutting from a turban of swirling clouds. "Remember, Mom, last night?"

Yes, I nodded, remembering the sight of the majestic mountain, lavender-purple against the late afternoon sky. A green sky, silhouetting the mountain and its crown of ice in jagged relief, its white crown visible, long into the encroaching night, like a lantern made of snow. Much later, when the flames of our campfire shot sparks of acacia wood into the darkness, rivaling for moments the constellations of Scorpio and the Little and Big Dipper, only then did the white of the snowcapped mountain dissolve into the African night.

The African night. Stars on the equator. "There are so many stars, Mother. I can't believe what I see." And Stephanie had sung, "Lucy in the sky with diamonds." She'd whispered in my ear, maybe so HE wouldn't hear, "God certainly has a lot of diamonds, diamonds, diamonds. . ."

"More beautiful in the sky than they could ever be on a woman," I whispered back.

We listened to the sounds of the savanna. The occasional bark of a zebra, the excitable screech of a baboon, the roar of a male lion. Beckoning his pride? Or roaring for the sheer pleasure of being alive?

That was all last night.

Now we were hungry, and our noses led us toward the smell of bacon and pancakes. Most of the food we ate was produced right here on the farm.

After breakfast we found Kilai, very black, wearing a very red shirt and standing by his very white horse, holding the two horses we were to ride. We mounted part-Arabian, polo-trained horses, able to turn on a dime. We rode English style, slowly, single file, through the high savanna grass, skirting the hills. Stephanie had ridden English saddle with me in Topanga Canyon several times. She fell off once when a rattle snake appeared and her horse reared. She broke her arm, but she had never shown any fear of horses or snakes after the incident.

Both of us now felt that nothing on earth could even remotely come close to this intense feeling of oneness with nature, the experience of sitting on a horse among herds of zebra and giraffe. We felt safe with Kilai and his gun, our protector. It was his job to guard against lions and to keep track of the many wild animals on the farm.

Suddenly he held out his hand. A warning. We stopped. A Black Mamba, coiled in the sand, raised its head and unhinged its jaw, to a show of magenta pink edged with pointed, razor-sharp teeth. A spray of venom flashed in the sun and landed near our horses' feet. The horses reared but didn't bolt. We stuck to our saddles. The black-green glistening snake, the most poisonous reptile in East Africa, flung itself into the high grass and disappeared. We remained motionless for a few more seconds, our hearts pounding. Then we rode on.

A few moments later Kilai greeted a reticulated giraffe, Charlie, like a long-lost friend. We wondered how he could tell this one was Charlie and not some other giraffe? The giraffes watched us. We watched the giraffes. They didn't run, they didn't walk, they undulated. We came very close, they batted their eyes, and their long straight lashes and puckered mouths gave them a "Clara Bow" look of surprise.

Steff said, "Hey, look at Charlie's lashes! He should be called Charlene."

And the zebras too, Grevy zebras here in the north of Kenya were different from the others we had seen. The Grevy, with its finely stenciled stripes and longer legs, looks like an aristocrat compared to the common zebra. A large male allowed us to approach just so near, then he signaled his females and he and his harem loped off.

It was magic, this ride through the savanna. Kilai explained to us that we could approach this close, because wild animals see only the horse. The human in the saddle is viewed as a sort of tumor on the horse's back. Grazing animals do not fear other grazers, making it possible to get much closer on horseback than would be possible on foot or in a jeep.

"Mom," Stephanie said, when we paused for a moment, "Thank you for taking me here. And thank you God, for making all of this so beautiful. I'm so lucky to be here."

I wanted to reach over and kiss her, but I didn't, fearing it might spook the horses.

The following day, David Craig took us to an area on his farm where Dr. Leaky had discovered hand axes of the Acheulian Period, the Lower Paleolithic period, about a million two hundred thousand years ago. The field was strewn with the uplifted remains of man's early tools. Stephanie picked one up, a piece of black obsidian, shaped like an oversized arrowhead, fitting easily into the palm of a hand.

Stephanie shook her head and asked, "This stone ax is one million years old?"

"Yes Stephanie. Some are even older."

"Wow!" She puzzled. "So—, somebody said that this is where it all began? Where we all came from?"

"That's right. All of us, all races. . .mankind began right here in East Africa." David took the hand ax Stephanie still held and put it back on the ground. We wound our way back between the stone tools used by our antecedents, and we walked with reverence.

Later, while we were sitting on canvas chairs in front of our tent, Stephanie looked up at the heavens and shook her head. "It's so unbelievable. The billions of stars, the beginning of earth and then. . .the beginning of man. The land feels so old and yet so new."

She grew pensive and then said, "And God made everything so beautiful. Mom, why do people hate each other? Why is there such a thing as racism? Why? We were all brothers once. Why can't we be aware of that and care for each other?"

How could I answer?

She leaned back in her chair, her eyes upon the stars. "Mom, now I know why you love Africa so much."

"Yes?"

"It is as if you can hear the earth breathe. You can hear its heartbeat." Her eyes closed and a smile played with her lips. "And, Mom, listen to the wind in the grass. . .listen!" She cupped her ear with her hand, "What is that sound?"

"Cicadas, Stephanie, a kind of grasshopper."

"The cicadas are singing a song, Mom. There must be millions of them, like the stars above. . .so many. . .everything moves and is alive. So, so, alive!"

And as she said this the roar of a lion shook the air.

Stephanie held her breath and reached for my hand. The reflection of the oil lamp's flame danced on her face. She pointed to shadows across a flat area, moving through the shoulder-high grass. Her hand tightened on mine. Neither of us spoke. I sensed her eyes, like mine, were straining to make out the shadowy forms. We listened. And then, against the clear starlit sky, animals appeared. One, two, three—more, six, seven Oryx were rising out of the depth of grass onto a hillock. Seeing them in profile, their two horns seemed welded into one. Stephanie let go of my hand, holding her mouth. Staring.

Unicorns, mythical creatures, as if created before our very eyes were mounting the hill and gently loping single file—outlined for a miraculous moment against the indigo sky—only to disappear again into the African night.

The wonders of Africa. Stephanie squeezed my hand and said, "Thank you, Mom. I'll never forget Africa."

And neither will I, Stephanie, neither will I.

Chapter Twenty

Back in the Land of Fear

Autumn 1983

The return from Africa threw us into a dark reality. In some bizarre way, I seemed to be experiencing things in reverse. Africa, the dark continent, had given me hope, and I had felt light and harmony. Back here, in our "white" world, I felt fear and an unlit void.

Stephanie picked up on my moods, and they mirrored in hers. My days were filled with visits to lawyers, with decisions to be made, and all of it made me feel apprehensive. I wished I had a savvy brother or cousin in California who could advise me as to what offers I should accept from Marvin. I knew so many lawyers and Steffi's grandfather Marvin's father, Poppy, the judge in Chattanooga, but they were all connected to my former family.

Stephanie saw very little of her father after we returned from Africa. I doubt he even read our letters. He never made any mention of them.

I tried to give Stephanie freedom to go out with her friends, but this created situations more dangerous than those we had encountered in Africa.

One day Stephanie went to the beach in Santa Monica with a friend from the Frostig Center and her mother. I was home when the phone rang. I could barely understand the foreign accented voice, crying, "It is not my fault, not my fault."

I finally recognized the speaker as Rachel's mother, the friend she had gone to the beach with. The woman sounded distraught. I grew more frantic by the minute, not being able to understand her clearly. *What? Did Stephanie have a seizure? Did she get hurt by a wave?* I knew my daughter was more sea otter than human in the water, and I ruled out drowning. But then, even though she had not had a seizure in many a year, there was always the possibility of one coming up suddenly. In the water this could be fatal.

Then I finally made sense of the woman's words: "She disappeared. She's gone." *Disappeared? When?* Around three. I checked the time. It was now nearly a quarter to five. I reprimanded the woman, "Why didn't you call me

153

sooner?" I was rude to her and sounded dictatorial, "You wait there. Don't you move. I'm on my way."

I reached Santa Monica in a ticket-deserving, speed-breaking twenty minutes. I knew where I would find them, and luckily found a parking slot. I raced across the sand to Rachel and her hysterical mother. They reported last seeing Stephanie, talking to a man in the water. He was aged about fortyish, balding. Then, suddenly—she was gone. How was that possible? Too furious to talk further, I marched across the sand to a lifeguard approaching in a vehicle, and explained the situation to him: Stephanie's handicaps, her reluctance to ask for help. I described my daughter, the blue-and-red patterned bikini she wore. I told the mother to stay put in that same spot in case Stephanie came back while the lifeguard and I were looking for her. Then he and I were off in the jeep, driving on the sand, looking for Steffi. At the next lifeguard tower the message was relayed to other lifeguards farther down the beach.

We had driven south from near the Santa Monica pier for perhaps one or two miles. Suddenly I spotted Stephanie! I yelled, pointing to her limping along near the water's edge, heading in the opposite direction from Rachel and her mother. The lifeguard stepped on the gas and then came to a sand-spraying halt. When I jumped from the jeep, she saw me, ran, fell into my arms, shaking, and crying. The sun hung low by then. She shivered with cold, clad in her flimsy bikini. I wrapped her in my sweater, held her while she sobbed.

The lifeguard interrupted, questioning Stephanie. "Was it a balding man who picked you up?"

"Yes," she answered, barely audible.

"Did he have a motorcycle?"

"Yes, a Honda. I think. And a camera." Her voice grew louder as she went on, "He said he wanted me to pose for him with his motorcycle—I'd make a good model." Turning to me she added, "Mom, he's a photographer for magazines."

The lifeguard frowned. "We know that guy. That's his line with women. We've had complaints. Better inform the police."

"But he didn't do anything, honest. Well. . .he tried to kiss me. I pushed him off. Yuck. He's *ug-ly*! And when he wanted to take my picture in his apartment, I told him flat out, no. I had to get back to my friends or they'd worry." Stephanie wiped her nose and eyes with my sweater, and we all climbed back into the jeep.

"So where were you all this time? You made us crazy with worry."

"He took me back to the beach, after he took a bunch of photos of me and his Honda."

"You went with him on his motorcycle like this? In a bikini? Stephanie, you—"

"Now Mom! Pleeeeze! That's all I had, this bikini. He did take me back. I tried to find Rachel, but she wasn't there. I couldn't find her, not her mother either. I looked for my towel, like you told me, the red towel. I didn't see it. Nothing. I walked and walked. . ." Tears ran down her face. Then she placed her foot on her knee to show me blisters forming.

"I guess you walked in the wrong direction," the lifeguard said.

I was still furious with Stephanie for having run off. But as upset as I was, I hugged her and kissed her, happy to have found her. My signals to her were as mixed as my thoughts concerning this episode. I was proud of her for not going to the man's apartment to be photographed, but on the other hand, she had described him as ugly. Would she have gone with him if he had been handsome?

I needed reinforcement. I hated asking for help, but in the end I called Marvin, hoping he would lecture her on what might have happened to her with this man.

I reached him. By his voice I could picture him shrugging off the entire incident. "She's okay, she's back home, isn't she? Let it be. Don't let her go to the beach unless you go along." I hung up—feeling weak, incompetent, and angry with myself for having asked for his help.

After this I did not allow Stephanie to go to the beach without me or my mother.

The Oaks in Ojai—a health spa about seventy miles north of Los Angeles—became my refuge. The Oaks kept me sane during these months of divorce proceedings. Stephanie often accompanied me. Exercise and yoga helped her arm and her right hand. Here, Steff made the acquaintance of Caryn Mandabach, a young television producer, who was kind to Stephanie and invited us to watch the filming of her new sitcom.

We were back in Los Angeles and were scheduled to see a taping of Caryn's show in the evening and later meet with the actors, Van Johnson and Madeline Kahn.

When I returned from an errand—I had driven the older car—I found the brown diesel Mercedes gone from where I had left it parked in front of our house.

Gloria came running, crying, "Estefani, she 'a take the key and she. . .gone."

"What do you mean? She took my car?"

"*Si.* She go, no say noathing, she go—"

Stephanie had a learners permit and taken a few driving lessons, but she certainly wasn't able to handle traffic at this stage. What made her do this? Where did she go? She had looked forward to going to the studio. She knew the taping was this evening. What now?

I called Caryn and told her what happened. I called Marvin and this time he showed concern. He came to the house with Judith. This was the first time that she'd set foot in my house, at least as far as I knew. Her presence added to the tension I already felt. Every nerve in my body felt hot and prickly, like electric wiring running right beneath the surface of my skin, wiring of 120 volts that was now charged with 240 volts.

They followed me into the kitchen. Marvin wanted to alert the police, but we both knew they would do little since Stephanie had not been declared incompetent. A psychiatrist had advised us not to take that drastic step, which would involve a court hearing where we would have to testify in Stephanie's presence that she was unable to act in her own interest. In short, we'd have to say that she was retarded. The doctor had warned that a court hearing would affect Stephanie's progress adversely. She must never think of herself as retarded.

It grew dark, and Marvin at last called the police. He explained that Stephanie was *severely retarded*. Retarded! Her father called her a severely retarded woman. The knife word. Now a double-bladed knife. I hoped he'd used this word in order for the police to help us.

Then he rubbed it in, this word. He turned to me and said, "Stephanie *is* retarded. You might as well admit it. *You* have a severely retarded daughter. Face it, Karin."

I left the kitchen. A lump grew big and bigger in my throat, but I wouldn't cry. Not in front of *them*. Then Marvin and Judy left to look for Stephanie. Not much time had passed before I heard the rumbling sound of the diesel-engine of my car roll into our driveway. Steffi rushed through the back door, fell into my arms, out of breath, her face flushed.

"Ah, Mom, gosh what a time I had. I got lost—"

"Where did you go? What made you—"

Marvin stormed in, grabbed her by the shoulders, held her at arm's length, and shook her. He forced her to look at him. "Stephanie, don't you ever do that again. Have you gone nuts? What made you do this?"

"Dunno," she answered with a shrug. She looked as if she were about to burst into tears, but then she turned to me and a half smile appeared beneath her wet lashes.

Judy explained, "We caught her, or rather, passed her as Steff went by us on Sunset, near the 405. We U-turned and followed. She drove like a maniac, screeching around the turns, she must have gone over ninety."

Stephanie narrowed her eyes and shot Judy a "drop-dead" look. "I did not!" She stomped her foot. "I drove carefully." After a pause she shrugged, saying, "But I did get lost."

Stephanie told of how she got onto the Santa Monica Freeway earlier on, then driving east—farther and farther—until she saw a sign, "Pomona." Here she remembered the fairgrounds and knew she'd gone too far and would have to turn around. She made a looping exit-entry, and got back onto the freeway, heading west. It was getting dark. She remembered to turn on her lights. After miles of driving she noticed the off ramp, "La Brea," a name that sounded familiar. Here she was confronted by several directional signs. She knew we lived north of Sunset, and thus she chose to go "North." When she finally reached Sunset, she headed west again. But by the time she came to our turnoff at Whittier, she failed to recognize the street. Perhaps she was too tired or too nervous. And so she overshot the right intersection and went all the way to the 405 at Sunset and Sepulveda, where quite correctly she made a U-turn for home.

I gave Marvin a defiant look, letting him know how smart I thought Stephanie was! And how wrong he was, thinking she was *severely* retarded.

But above all, Stephanie had been lucky. We were lucky. Had she turned south on La Brea, she might have ended up in gang territory. A young girl, without money, without identification, in a luxury car.

I exhaled with relief. Stephanie was home. I held her tight for a very long time. It was good to feel her warmth, smell her hair, my child, safe again. But I worried. What was this new "breaking-out" spirit possessing her, that had made her take off with a stranger on the beach, and then again tonight in the car? Was it a yearning to be independent, free to go as she wished? More than anything I would like for Stephanie to enjoy freedom; but her freedom had to be limited. Sadly, our urban jungle was not a safe place for her.

A few weeks later I was on my way to pick her up from the dentist. When I turned the corner I saw her already standing on the street, waving excitedly.

"Mom, guess what?" she blurted out as she climbed into the car. "Mom, I have a job!" What she said didn't register. I flushed with anger when I said, "Steff, why weren't you waiting for me inside? What were you doing out on the street?"

"Mom, listen! You never listen. I've got a job. Me, your daughter Stephanie Diane Finell, is going to work in the Swiss Bakery."

"Okay." I pulled over into a driveway to turn around. "Okay, now, go slow. What's this about a Swiss Bakery?"

"See the sign?" She pointed to a large "Help Wanted" in the window of the bakery on the corner. "I was done early, and I had some money. I thought I'd get one of their yummy chocolate chip cookies. The really big ones. And then I saw the sign. Well. . .I smiled at the owner, and told him I would like to work. That's all." She sounded chipper and crinkled her perky nose. "He gave me the job. I start tomorrow."

"Stephanie, you—" I was about to say *you can't*, but then I bit my lip.

Stephanie guessed what I was thinking and said, "Yes, I can. Let me try! Okay, Mom?"

The next day I took her to the bakery. She wore the required white blouse and dark skirt, while the shop would supply the apron and a little white cap. I helped her fill out forms. Stephanie told the owner that she had suffered from equine encephalitis (he'd probably never heard of that disease, as I had not before Stephanie got ill) and as a result was slightly handicapped. She showed him her right hand and told him it was partially paralyzed. This did not seem to discourage him.

When I spoke to him and tried to make him aware of her limitations, he told me not to worry. "With that smile, your daughter will sell more pastries in one day than the others do in a week."

When I picked her up after her first day of work, she flashed *me* this big Stephanie smile. A moment later she cried. Stephanie liked the work and the other women, most of them my age, who were kind and helpful. But there had been several mishaps. Trying to balance a creamy pie, she was unable to maneuver it into its pink cardboard box. It slid to the floor. The women helped Stephanie with mopping up the mess, saying, "It's okay, it's your first day." But later her paralyzed right hand did not obey her when folding the pink boxes or lining them with wax paper. She bravely promised, "Tomorrow I'll do better."

Several days went by. Then one day around noon, the owner phoned and, with a flood of apologies, asked me to come early and pick Stephanie up. When I entered through the glass door, I found her sitting at one of the small iron-footed marble tables with a half-eaten strawberry tart in front of her, crying and eating. Then she saw me and her eyes brightened. She handed me an envelope, saying, "Open it, Mom, my first paycheck!"

The owner seemed genuinely sad and acted somewhat guilty about letting Stephanie go.

"Stephanie's embarrassed by her. . .hmm, handicaps. She knows how to hide them, for a while at least," I said. "It was nice of you to hire her. Thanks for trying."

"And her smile," he rhapsodized. "Her smile. . .it lit up my bakery."

Time passed. Our first holidays went by without Marvin and then the year of 1984 began. Marvin and I were still not divorced. My life in Beverly Hills was one of constant torment, where every little thing reminded me of our former life as a family, of our former happiness. I wanted to escape again and decided to go on a lengthy trip to the Himalayas, trekking in Ladakh, Western Tibet, and to visit Buddhist lamasteries—monasteries. I hoped to find a new insight into life, an illumination, if you will. A trip too strenuous—and medically speaking, too isolated and therefore dangerous—for Stephanie to take. Stephanie flew to Guadalajara to spend those months with Carmen and Alonso, who had declared Stephanie their gringa daughter, while their two sons and two daughters treated her indeed like a sister. Stephanie was eager to see her Mexican family again. For two months we went our separate ways.

When I returned home, I was eager to see my daughter again, having missed her those many weeks. To my surprise, she was not at all ready to return from Mexico. Carmen pleaded, and I allowed her to remain and attend yet another fiesta, another wedding, another christening. When she finally did come home, I hardly recognized her. Carmen had taken her to get a new and stylish haircut, her clothes were clinging and sexy, all in all I was amazed at this sophisticated young lady walking toward me from the Mexicana Airlines gate at the Los Angeles airport.

In September 1984, Gloria, our housekeeper, married and left us. We found a replacement in Aida, also from Guatemala, ten years older than Gloria. In time Aida became a second mother to Stephanie.

"Mom, do you know that Aida's husband left her? And he left her for his. . . his first cousin? Like Dad and—"

"Really? She told you this?"

"Yes, and listen to this. It's so weird. She has a daughter, Patti, and she's as upset as I am about her father dumping her."

"Your father didn't dump you, Stephanie. He left *me*. You must remember that."

"He *dumped* me, Mom. I never ever see him alone. Always with Judy. That—"

"Hush, Stephanie. He's living with her now. Please, you must accept that he's gone. But he loves you. I know that."

Stephanie sucked in her lips, shook her head. "Funny, he doesn't show it. . . And you know what else?"

"With your father?"

"No, with Aida. She also grew up with just her mother and her grandmother. Exactly like you! Her parents were also divorced. . .gee, that's so bizarre, you and Aida—"

"Like parallel lives. You understood all she told you? Your Spanish really improved in Guadalajara."

"I like speaking Spanish. Alonso calls it *spanglish*."

Early in the fall, while at the Santa Monica beach with my mother, Stephanie met Raul. When I picked her up from Mother's, Stephanie gushed about how handsome he was.

When I met Raul, I agreed. He was tall, good-looking, twenty-one years old, with black anthracite eyes, burning like dry ice. Stephanie fell "in love" with this young man, but after a while she became skeptical. He loved guns and took her with him to target practice. "Boring—" Stephanie reported. He did not act as romantic as his looks promised but, rather, liked to parachute and drive his father's sports car at more than a hundred miles per hour.

At the movies, Stephanie found a wallet. Raul snatched it, fought Stephanie for it, and took all the money, about ninety dollars. Stephanie was making a scene, arguing loudly, trying to turn the wallet over to the box office. Raul shook her to quiet her. She was silent after the rough treatment, while Raul threw the wallet in the trash. Stephanie came home that evening in an irate mood but would not tell me the reason for her anger. A week later, after Raul bought a handgun with the money, she told me the story of the wallet.

I had begun to worry about Stephanie's relationship with Raul. He professed to love her, and he talked about marriage after he graduated from the flight mechanics school he attended. But something about him troubled me, something I couldn't put my finger on. He came from an educated family, though I felt his Argentinean father imposed too many restrictions and rules (among them attending Mass twice on Sundays), while Raul still suffered from the death of his German American mother. Barely a year had passed since his mother died of cancer. Perhaps I could excuse his often irrational behavior as the result of unresolved grief. But still, there was something else, something intangible. I had met enough students at Stephanie's special schools to intuit if a person was afflicted with problems. His possessiveness frightened Stephanie. His eyes could become distant and cruel. One day, in a fit of unprovoked jealousy, he hit her in the middle of her face with his fist, bloodying her nose.

"Out! Get out of this house! Right now, get out!" I heard Stephanie scream. Then I heard the clicking of footsteps running down the stairs, followed by the slam of the front door. That was the last time we saw Raul.

Chapter Twenty-One

The Black Knight

Enter Rick, the Black Knight

Clad in black leather, he appeared out of nowhere on his black Harley David-son steed, and he caused Stephanie's reason to fly off, on the draft of wind, the wind created by riding at top speed through our nearby canyons.

How she loved the feeling of freedom on the motorcycle—and fell for the allure of the forbidden. And he, full of testosterone, appeared like a remedy to her disappointment with the virginal Raul. But of course, she didn't tell me any of this. Not in the beginning.

Rick had taken a drive into the movie-star-map section of Beverly Hills where we lived. He stopped his shiny motorcycle and began talking to Stepha-nie. That day she wore a red T-shirt and white shorts, showing tanned and shapely legs and walking Duke, the Irish setter we had recently picked up from the pound.

Stephanie's limitations were not visible, and sadly, her surging hormones hampered her ability to judge men. Also, had she not been brain-injured, she never would have spoken more than a few words with Rick.

These rides were dangerous for her in many ways. While balancing on the motorbike, she was holding on to Rick with her paralyzed right hand—fraught with danger. But worst of all, she did not wear a helmet.

Stephanie began lying, and since I was accustomed to her former truthful-ness, did not suspect anything was amiss. But I did wonder why Stephanie suddenly showed such enthusiasm for walking the dog. I should have real-ized it was strange that neither Duke nor Stephanie ever looked tired when they returned. No wonder. She leashed the poor dog to a lamppost about a block down the street (opposite of Barbra Streisand's house on Carolwood Drive), while Stephanie was off, rocketing through the rises and valleys of Holmby Hills and Bel Air—up and over Mulholland Drive, zooming down to the San Fernando Valley and back to Brentwood, and on and on. All without any clothing to protect her in case Rick took a spill. While Reckless Rick rode encased in black leather and a helmet.

He swore Stephanie to secrecy. But to keep silent about these adventures was too much to ask of her. And finally she bubbled over with talk. She told me that he lived with his uncle, and that the uncle had bought him the Harley.

I worried deeply about this enigma, this Rick. He said he was twenty-two years old and had left high school before graduation. He had worked as a roofer. This man he called *uncle* had met him who-knows-where and tried to play Professor Higgins as in *My Fair Lady*. Only Rick was no Eliza Doolittle. The uncle bought him suitable clothes and took him on a Caribbean cruise. The uncle was Anglo, but Rick's high cheekbones, his narrow nose and full lips, his black, short-cropped kinky hair and café-au-lait skin, his slanted eyes, all indicated he was a mix of races. He had an athlete's body and long legs, and he might have been considered handsome had it not been for his lascivious grin that displayed stained teeth, protruding fan-like, almost horizontally.

When I opened the door, and Steff introduced him to me, his expression was sly and cunning. We shook hands, and he held onto my hand much too long. His hand was damp, and I wanted to drop it. He held on to my hand, tight. His squinting gaze stripped me naked. I finally was able to jerk my hand loose, itching to wipe the leer off his face.

When I objected to her going out with Rick, she called me a racist. I begged Marvin to intervene, to have a father-daughter talk with her.

His answer was curt, "Sorry, I'm going to leave for Europe in two days. I don't have time."

Steven, at six foot two inches and built like a football player, was my only hope to intimidate Rick. They met, and Steven told Rick to stay away from his sister. The result was that Stephanie screamed at her brother and labeled him a racist, too. From then on she met Rick in secret. A few weeks later she disappeared.

I called the uncle. My suspicions were confirmed. Stephanie and Rick had run off. Rick and his Harley were gone. "Don't worry," the uncle tried to calm me. "They'll be back when they run out of money."

Marvin was out of town. Should I call the police? Stephanie was a month short of twenty-one. I knew the police would do nothing. I spent a terrified, sleepless night.

In the morning the phone rang, a collect call from Las Vegas. It was Rick. "We're married," he said. A shooting pain went from my head to my heart then moved to my stomach, causing waves of nausea. I leaned against the door frame to keep from falling.

"We don't have any money," Rick went on. "Guess we'll sleep on the street. Or. . ." he drew out his words. "Can you wire us two hundred dollars? Can you do that?"

"Let me talk to Stephanie," I said.

"She isn't here right now." Then his voice grew threatening. "Tell me *now,* are you going to send us the money or not?"

"Listen, Rick." I tried to stall him while my thoughts raced on, working out a solution. "I don't have the money to send by wire. Wait. . .I have a cousin in Vegas. I'll try to get hold of him. Maybe he can meet you, bring some money. Call me back in an hour."

We hung up.

Social workers had warned that something like this might happen. Girls and women with head trauma have a difficult time restraining their sexuality, and since they are not discriminating, they become easy prey for unscrupulous men. Since Stephanie was not declared incompetent, there was nothing any agency could do to protect her. I protected her, but I also had allowed her to experience a degree of freedom, to experience life as it presented itself. I regretted not being able to lock her into her room.

I remembered a story from my mother's life. When she was Stephanie's age, she fell in love with a pilot who wanted to train her to be a wing-walker and move from town to town to perform in air shows, which were popular at that time. Mother was a daredevil and wanted to learn to fly, but my grandfather, a stern lawyer, discovered their plan and locked Mother into her room for a week. Until the young pilot left town. I could not do this to Stephanie.

Instead I got on the phone to my cousin Richard in Las Vegas. Richard, a retired Air Force colonel raised on a ranch in Utah, now rode to the rescue in the reliable tradition of the Old West. This was our plan: I would fly to Las Vegas, Richard and I would meet Stephanie and Rick in a specified hotel where I would try to convince Stephanie to fly back home with me.

Later in the afternoon, Richard and I pushed through the glass doors to the bar of the Frontier Hotel. At the bar sat Rick, and next to him, Stephanie. She wore her red leather jacket paired with clothes I didn't recognize. My knees buckled, seeing her like this. Her bare legs were wrapped around a barstool. She wore the shortest of tight skirts and high-heeled red boots. Her hair looked unwashed and stringy. Her normally fresh and pretty face looked disfigured by caked-on makeup. For one brief instant I wished I could become invisible and crawl out of the room before she would see me, but no, I was fully aware of the danger she was in. I had to rescue her. Hideous thoughts chased through my mind. Why did he let her dress like this? What would he force her to do if I hadn't come?

I took a deep breath and grabbed Richard's arm a little tighter. We went to where she sat, sipping a Piña Colada. She looked up at me, her eyes dull and glazed. No hugs. She merely waved her drink at me, saying, "Hi, Mom, I'm married."

I bit my lip, fighting tears and fighting my desire to grab her and hug her. I sounded distant when I said, "Yes. Rick told me. Where's your ring?"

"Rick will buy me one later. We didn't have any money."

"But you have money for cocktails in the afternoon?"

"Chill out, Mom. Don't bitch at me."

Who is this girl? This is not my daughter. She never talks to me like this.

Earlier, Rick had noticed us when we first entered the bar. Seeing me with Richard must have shocked him, for he rocked back on his bar stool but caught himself before it tipped over. His mouth gasped for air like a carp out of water. But he was smart enough to know he was at a disadvantage and had to play our game. For now.

The four of us talked over dinner, and by then I knew Stephanie would not come home with me alone. "Now that you're married, you can stay at my house for a night or two," I told them, trying to buy time. Rick realized there would be no money from me at this point and was afraid I might involve the police. I had lied to Rick out of desperation and made him believe I had that option in view of Stephanie's disabilities. Richard took us to the airport. I hugged him and thanked him for being there in this time of need. Then, Stephanie, Rick, and I took the next flight back to LAX.

The following day Stephanie accompanied Rick to Los Angeles General Hospital trauma center, where he was to be treated for a previous, by now infected, dog bite.

While Rick and Stephanie were gone, I searched her belongings for proof of the marriage. I felt rotten doing this, never having snooped in anyone's personal effects before, but I *had* to know. I found no marriage certificate. Nothing. *Nada.* The closest thing I found was the brochure of a wedding chapel. I called their number on the slim chance they still remembered if they married a couple as dissimilar as Stephanie and Rick.

"They didn't get married," a woman's voice told me. "The girl didn't have any ID, she looked so young, so innocent. Like fifteen. . .maybe less. We wouldn't marry them."

I packed Rick's bags.

Stephanie was in tears when they came home, telling me about the many people crowding into the emergency room, among them a man who carried his severed hand in a shoebox, pleading to see a doctor immediately to have the hand reattached to the bloody, bandaged stump of his arm.

I took Stephanie aside. She noticed from my expression that something was wrong. I told her that I knew Rick and she were not married. Her mouth opened wide, partially in astonishment, or as if to say something with no words coming forth. I told her to listen.

"Stephanie, it's no use. Never mind how I found out. You cannot live here with Rick. If you want to live with him, you are free to go, but you won't get one penny from me. Not from your father either. Rick will have to find work and support you."

"He can't, Mom." Her nose clogged up, she whispered, "He's poor. And now his motorcycle's stuck in Vegas. And he's got that dog bite." Then she yelled, "Aren't you the one who's always sorry for poor people?"

"Yes. People who have problems. . .he's not incapable of working. His uncle told me—"

"His uncle is *not* his uncle!" Stephanie stomped her foot. "And once his Harley is back, he's taking it away. He's really mean. Just because he's jealous that Rick's with me. He won't let us stay with him either. So where do you want us to go, Mom, huh, where?"

I knew I was playing a dangerous game. I might lose. But I stayed firm. "You can go wherever you want with Rick," I said. "But you can't stay here with him. Stephanie, I love you and I forgive you for running away, but if you want to live here, you'll have to promise me, you won't see Rick again. No one knows the future. Perhaps he'll turn his life around. Then we'll see about you and Rick. But for now, he must go."

"Mom. . .? I love you." She ran to me and put her arms around me. After a pause, still testing, she asked, "Sure?"

"Yes, Stephanie. I'm very sure. He must leave."

Stephanie let out a deep sigh. Almost as though she were relieved I had made up her mind for her. She again spoke of the man with the severed hand, the mass of people crowding into the emergency room. "I can't live that way, Mom. I can't live the way Rick wants me to live. Perhaps it's best—"

Then I confronted Rick. Stephanie sat very still with her eyes fixed onto the swaying queen palm outside our window. She didn't look up, did not utter one word. Only when Rick reached the door, ready to leave, and asked, "Steffi, don't you want to come with me?" did she slowly raise her head. "No Rick, it won't work," she said. "It's best if you go."

I took him to the nearest bus stop, gave him some money to get out of our neighborhood, and returned home. I was still trembling, though I felt I had won a victory.

I took Stephanie to Dr. Silton, the ob/gyn who had brought her into this world, to have her checked out for any STD she might have picked up through Rick. The report came back that she was healthy. But Dr. Silton cautioned me about the probability that now, since she was sexually active, she might get pregnant. I told him I would watch her and see to it that she had no opportunity to be with a man, but he only smiled.

"She is a young woman," he said, "the only way she will be safe is with birth control pills or with a copper spiral inserted in her uterus. Given her condition, she would be forgetful and couldn't be trusted to take her pills with regularity.

The spiral is the best solution." I inquired further into this suggested birth control method and was told it was safe, and in her case it made sense. A copper spiral was inserted, and Stephanie did not complain.

On November 10, for Stephanie's twenty-first birthday, Uncle Bud, and his new wife, Shirley, invited Stephanie to fly to Las Vegas. I put her on the plane, and they sent a limo to pick her up. The irony of it. Now she would experience a different Las Vegas, an elegant room in Caesar's Hotel, and urbane people who celebrated the occasion of Bud Seretean receiving the highest award the carpet industry bestowed.

Shirley told me that Stephanie regaled the guests at their table with tales of Africa, the lion kill she had witnessed, and she told them about a Maasai warrior who wanted to buy her for fifty cows. Shirley and Bud were impressed with how she entertained their sophisticated guests. They said I should be very proud of her, because she gave the impression to have matured so beautifully. It seemed that no one noticed she was not a young woman going to college since she acted so self-assured. I smiled when I got the report, thinking that the trip to Africa had helped her to learn and grow. But it had not made her mature enough to realize that a man like Rick lived a world apart from any of our relatives or friends. I kept worrying whether she would ever learn.

When she came back from Las Vegas, now twenty-one, I found a curriculum for her that promised to teach independence. She attended daily classes at an Easter Seals program near downtown Los Angeles to prepare her for her goal: to live on her own. In the beginning, I took her and picked her up, but the therapists suggested that I allow her to be more independent and take the bus. She boarded the same bus every morning at the corner of Whittier and Wilshire, opposite from her first school, El Rodeo. Ron, one of her co-students (a sweet-faced man) took the same bus. In many ways he was more developmentally disabled than Stephanie, but he did not get lost, and I felt Stephanie was safe in his company.

A month or two into the program my phone rang. The director was on the line. "Stephanie didn't arrive in school today," she said. "Ron told us she got off the bus with a man she knew. Would you know who this might be?"

I checked the time. It was ten o'clock, and Stephanie's classes started at nine. *Where was she? With Rick? Oh please, not Rick!* The room spun around me. Then I splashed cold water on my eyes and grabbed the car keys.

I drove to the school to question Ron. "Yes," he stammered. "He did have weird teeth. . .Stephanie acted like she was happy to see him. She said she was going to have coffee and a doughnut. The guy would take her to school later."

It was Rick.

Rick's "uncle" was my only hope. If he was jealous of Stephanie, would he not help me to get her away from Rick? I guessed right. When I called him, he was as upset as I was that Rick had run off again with Stephanie. He told me that Rick expected a settlement sum of twenty-five thousand dollars from his attorney for the dog bite. Rick would pick the money up—most likely in the morning when the bank first opened—in the same building where the lawyer's office was located. He gave me the name of the bank and the address.

There was something wrong with this California "justice." Rick had been bitten by a watchdog doing its duty, while climbing over a garden wall with dubious intent.

I set the alarm clock, making sure I had plenty of time for coffee and cornflakes and time to collect my thoughts before this encounter. I drove to the bank at the corner of Crescent and Wilshire, not far from our house. I arrived fifteen minutes before the bank opened. I waited, and waited, with my back turned to the building's entrance door, pretending to read the names on the directory. I kept reading them over and over.

Then a man pushed through the doors. Rick. Rick alone, without Stephanie. He didn't see me when he entered the bank. I watched him through the glass partition, watched him receive a wad of cash, and watched him cramming it into his pocket. *Oh my God!* Now he turned, coming toward me. I stepped forward and said, "Hello."

Rick was well aware of the change in our situation. After all, he now held the trump card: Stephanie. And he had twenty-five thousand dollars in his pocket. He was quite willing to have a cup of coffee with me, and "talk things over."

In the end, he told me where she was. His friend, a janitor, had allowed Rick and Steff to sleep on the roof of the Comstock Building on Wilshire, a mile or two from our house. Later Stephanie told me how romantic it was to sleep under the stars with the city lights twinkling below.

When we parted that morning, I persuaded Rick to bring Stephanie home for a visit. The hours ticked by. At last I heard a car drive up our street, and watching through the sheer curtains, I saw a cherry-red automobile stop in front of our house. There she was, Stephanie, hopping out from behind the wheel and rushing up the brick stairs.

"Mom, Mom, see this car? Rick bought me it. He bought me this car!"

Not *Sorry, Mom, for running away again.* No. Rick had bought her a shiny red car.

"Stephanie, you don't know how to drive."

"Yes I do. I drove all the way to Pomona, remember?"

Rick added, "She has her driver's permit with her. I'll teach her."

Stephanie skipped upstairs. I heard her dashing around in her room.

"Rick, I want to talk with you," I said, grabbing his elbow and steering him into the kitchen's breakfast nook. "You have some money now. If you love Stephanie, you can make a new start." I indicated for him to take a seat, while pouring fresh coffee. He looked at me stone-faced, dead-eyed, while I went on with my desperate pitch. "Try to get a job, Rick. Invest a little money, maybe in this roofing business where you worked before. Turn your life around. Stephanie will still be here, but don't force anything. Maybe you can come here and continue to give her driving lessons. . .take her out to see a movie. I won't be against that. The only thing I have against you is. . .is that you are. . ." My anger and disgust were mounting. I had to stop myself from saying something I'd regret. Taking a deep breath, I said, "You know you don't think of tomorrow. I think you'd be happier if you had a regular job. You'd make Stephanie happy."

"Okay, okay. We'll see." His foot tapped a faster and faster beat on the floor. Getting up he said, "But she's happy right now."

Steffi burst into the room, carrying her suitcase. She shook her head to say *No*, at the mention of coffee and cake, blew me a kiss, and dragged Rick out of the house into the shiny red car.

The police refused to search the roof of the apartment building when I reported her missing. I could have slapped myself for not acting sooner. When she appeared with the suitcase, I should have grabbed it from her and if need be wrestled with her to get the learner's permit from her handbag. Why was I trying to be civil with that Rick? If need be I could have called the police then, they would have come to my house and their appearance alone would have scared him. Again I faced the same quandary: the police would not act since Stephanie had not been declared incompetent. Marvin acted nonchalant, no reason to worry, he said. I could not understand his aloof behavior, he who had loved his little Snorg so very much. I told him I was afraid Stephanie could get married now, since she had her learner's permit with her, stating her age. Again he said, "Don't worry about it. Let's see what happens next." I felt like choking him over the telephone.

The next day Rick called from Las Vegas to announce that they were indeed married. This time it was real. I informed her father. "We'll just have to wait until she comes back and then have the marriage annulled," he said.

"But. . .I think we should go to court and have her declared incompetent."

"Maybe we can find another reason. But first she has to be back."

"What if she doesn't come back? What if he infects her with some horrible disease? And I think he's prostituting himself with this uncle. What if he's a pimp? What will he make her do when they run out of money?"

"You're very premature with these worries. Just be calm and wait, she'll be back."

I couldn't be calm. I wanted to bang my head against the wall, have a "tizzy-fit" as Stephanie called other children's tantrums. Marvin was an attorney, Marvin had connections. *Why wouldn't he help me? Help his own daughter for Christ's sake.* This time I was not a strong "German girl." I couldn't sleep without taking a Valium. In the morning when I climbed out of bed, I had to wade through a wad of wet tissues. When I looked in the mirror, my reflection shocked me. My eyes were ghoulish, puffy and red.

Perhaps the uncle would help me. After all, he too had an interest in getting Rick to come back to him. I didn't relish visiting him, but I felt I had to. This time he revealed more of Rick's checkered background. A warrant was out for him in Texas for attempting to pimp his twelve-year-old half sister to an older man in Dallas. I felt sick to my stomach when I heard this. I had guessed at these things in Rick's past without knowing any particulars.

"Now he has money," the uncle said, shaking his head, "He acts the big shot. But the money won't last long. Soon they'll be back."

Postcards from Stephanie and Rick began to arrive. The first from Albuquerque, and then another from Texas. It surprised me that Rick would travel to that state where a warrant was out for his arrest. Later a card arrived from Salt Lake City followed by one from Yellowstone. It astounded me how Rick and Stephanie crisscrossed the country.

It was early May, and they'd been gone for over six weeks. The phone rang a few minutes before 2:00 p.m., a collect call from Rick in Flagstaff, Arizona. He said he'd been arrested at 3:00 a.m. for speeding. Later I found out it was also for obstructing the peace and for possession of illegal drugs. He was held in jail. He asked me to bail him out, so he could "rescue" Stephanie.

"Where is Stephanie?"

"She's with some friends of mine. She's okay."

"Then why say rescue her?"

"She's gonna be lonely and scared without me. So will you please send the bail money?"

I remained silent for a moment. Then I muttered something while taking down the telephone number of the bail person. I called. After the first ring a woman answered. Good, I thought, maybe she's a mother and will have empathy. I explained to her that Stephanie was a victim of this man. I hated to have to explain her encephalitis, her brain damage, over and over again. But I had to let the woman know Stephanie's background and why I hadn't involved the police.

The woman sounded like a kind person and understanding. She gave me the name of the sheriff on the case. I called him. I told him the same story and asked him to please not let Rick go free until Stephanie was in my care again. He promised. The sheriff gave me the name and address of the motel where the Salvation Army had paid for two nights of Stephanie's stay.

I called Hugi, Stephanie's friend from ballet school.

"Sure, I'll come," she said. "It'll just take me a minute to get ready. I'll be in front of the house, waiting."

Soon Hugi and I were on the plane bound for Phoenix. We wolfed down our dinner, I rented a car, and we drove to Flagstaff. Although it was May, it was bitingly cold at seven thousand feet altitude when we arrived in the middle of night. We found the location of the modest motel with some difficulty, woke up the manager, and were shown to Stephanie's room.

There we found her asleep on a rumpled bed, surrounded by garish neon-colored carnival animals. Rick must have been a good shot to have won so many stuffed lions, bears, and who knows what.

"Mom. . .? Is that you, Mom? Who? Hugi? You?"

"Yes, Stephanie," Hugi and I answered simultaneously, while I had reached Stephanie's bed and was hugging my newly found daughter. "Get up, we're taking you to another hotel. Please, up, up."

"Wait for Rick—" she mumbled.

"Nix waiting for Rick," said Hugi. "He's in jail. You get yourself together, girl. Pronto. We're outa this dump."

Slowly Stephanie crept out of bed. She was still fully dressed in jeans and sweater. Stephanie swayed as if drunk, her eyes were dull and clouded. I was afraid she might have had a seizure. Hugi suspected drugs, and perhaps she was right.

Halfway through the door Stephanie stopped and grabbed a magenta giraffe. I clasped her shoulder. She let go of the giraffe, a sad little smile on her face. I believed she understood, even in her peculiar frame of mind, that we were taking her back to her former life, which would not include reminders of her most recent escapade.

The three of us checked into a Best Western motel, and I fell asleep, feeling the soft warmth of Stephanie's breath on my face.

The next morning we went to the sheriff's station to ask for Rick's car keys. We explained that Stephanie's personal items were in the car and we had to have the keys. He handed them to me reluctantly, only after I promised to bring them straight back.

While looking for Rick's car Stephanie sobbed and complained that Rick had sold *her* car and bought this older jeep, with a stick shift, which she could not drive. The shiny red car was history, the first of her dreams with Rick to shatter.

Stephanie, again dressed in jeans and sweater was warm, but Hugi and I were shivering, actually freezing. We had not anticipated that it would be this cold. I wore a silk dress I'd worn earlier in Los Angeles, and a light jacket, and now my bare feet in sandals sloshed through melting snow, while gritty ice particles clung to my naked toes.

I shuddered with disgust when I opened the jeep's door, having to dig through Rick's paraphernalia. The smell of the dirty laundry nauseated me. I took only one or two items of Stephanie's clothing and left the rest. But I had to search for Stephanie's address book. Eureka! I found it. I did not want Rick to contact any of our relatives to extort money, which he had tried during their previous adventure. That time, Rick had called Gammy and Poppy, as well as Aunt Farol. Luckily, no one believed him. They told him to have Stephanie herself get in touch if she was in trouble.

Before we left Flagstaff, I returned Rick's car keys to the sheriff and asked the kindly man to please call and warn me when they were releasing him.

The sheriff in Flagstaff kept his promise and phoned after Rick's release. I called our Westec Security Alarm Service and hired a guard in case Rick came to the house. Nine hours after the call from Flagstaff, our doorbell rang. The uniformed guard, hand on his gun in holster, opened the front door. He served Rick the restraining order we'd obtained earlier from the court. That was the last time we saw Rick.

A week later Stephanie complained of abdominal pain and began to bleed more heavily than during a normal menses. Again I took her to Dr. Silton. After he examined her, the folds in his face deepened, while the corners of his lips moved downward in disgust. He informed me that the copper spiral had been removed. Maybe forcibly. When I questioned Stephanie later, she broke down crying. I had a hard time understanding what she was saying.

"Mom, Rick said he loved me and wanted a baby from me." She wiped her nose with the back of her hand, then reached for a Kleenex and blew hard. "He said it wouldn't hurt, but it did." She blew her nose again. "He tried to take that thingy out. Boy, it really hurt. I told him to stop, it hurt so bad. He smacked me. 'Shut up,' he yelled. 'Just shut the hell up.' I tried to stop crying, but just then he turned and threw something in the trash."

I held her tight. We sat silent. There were no words, no words. . .Stephanie shook, reliving the event, and I stroked her hair, repeating, "Shh. . .all is well now—"

I could not believe this monster Rick, and when I too shook, it was with rage. *What should I do? What could I do?* I did not want to go to court and press charges. That would mean confronting Rick and letting him back into our lives. So I forced myself to shut the book on the chapter of Rick.

After a few weeks, I saw changes in Stephanie that made me believe that she no longer thought of Rick, that she had adjusted to her former life again. Yet there was the constant fear that another man might take advantage of her. Men were drawn to her. And she was so trusting. The newspapers were full of stories of men preying on women of sound mind and judgment. What chance did Stephanie have, who looked at the world from the perspective of a trusting child? If I wanted Stephanie to experience love and life, what price would she have to pay?

Soon Stephanie was radiant, shiny, and sparkling again. I thought of gold, how mud cannot cling to it but rinses off immediately. And a line by William Blake came to mind:

"The soul of sweet delight / can ne'er be defiled."

There was one coda to the story of Raul. Early in April, Mother by chance ran into Raul in a Santa Monica market. He told her he had graduated from the flight mechanics school, and as soon as he got a job, he would be in a position to marry Stephanie. Mother shook her head and said, "Sorry, you're too late. Stephanie has eloped to Las Vegas."

It was Raul's sister who discovered the body. Returning home from work, she found the white chenille bedspread drenched in red, and Raul's body slumped on her bed. The gun purchased with the money "found" in the wallet, had dropped from his limp hand, a single bullet had pierced his skull.

When Stephanie heard of Raul's death, she trembled and hid her face in her arms. I was afraid she'd have a seizure.

We both wept for a life not fully lived.

Chapter Twenty-Two

New Beginnings

The horror show of Rick faded into a blank screen. Marvin hired an attorney, and Stephanie and I went to court to have the Las Vegas marriage annulled. We were lucky: Rick did not contest and did not appear in court.

Our house was on the market again and I kept busy making it presentable for the many "Open Houses" we had. I can't count the many gladioli I bought for the downstairs rooms, and the many cinnamon muffins we wound up eating after the potential buyers left. I fell for the real estate agent's advice to brew fresh coffee and bake muffins to make the house smell homey. In retrospect that was silly—and shame on me for not recognizing it. Most of the would-be-buyers were in the movie business, or they were so well-off they were not looking for "Little House on the Prairie" hominess. The realtor liked coffee and cinnamon muffins, and I willingly went along with the advice because the "coziness" appealed to me, and Stephanie and I too liked to munch on the muffins.

The few serious buyers usually scheduled private appointments during the week. I left the house on those days. Once I was still in the house when I overheard a scratchy-voiced woman, her voice shrilling to the downstairs, complain about the lack of a special cedar-lined closet for furs. "Doesn't she have any minks and sables?" I heard her ask. And though I had some good furs, it no longer felt right to me to wear them.

The worst were the many curious, who just wanted to see how people in our part of town lived. After a small silver frame from the Civil War, a present from my father in-law who had found it in an antique shop in Chattanooga, had disappeared, I made sure a friend or my mother were present during these "Open House" days.

I spent my days taking writing classes at UCLA Adult Education. I wrote a screenplay, but during this turmoil in my life I found it difficult to concentrate. Then there was Stephanie. There was no program for her at this time.

She expressed an interest in flower arrangements. I enrolled her in a class in Santa Monica City College. Again, I shuttled her back and forth. Her progress pleased me, as she did extremely well in her class, especially considering her right hand was paralyzed. On those days when my mother picked her up and brought her home, Stephanie reported that she had inherited the talent of flower arranging from grandma. There was truth in that. Mother had always arranged flowers as a painter would, using blossoms according to color and combining them with branches from citrus trees or autumn-tinged shrubs, even using ornamental vegetables in her arrangements. Now mother and Stephanie together created some exotic bouquets for my "Open House" days.

Stephanie exercised in the Beverly Hills Gym with me, and I took her ice-skating in Santa Monica. I found a class where they taught her skills such as how to use an electric stove, how to change linens on a bed, and how to complete simple tasks of housekeeping. We went to the library together where I taught her how to use the index files to find the books she wanted to read.

Books presented a problem for her. She would forget what she had read on page 1 when she came to page 2, requiring her to read the same text over and over, until some of it became ingrained in her memory.

Stephanie and I visited Dr. Marianne Frostig in her condo in Santa Monica, when she mentioned Work Training Programs, Inc. A look of motherly concern crossed her face when she mentioned that Stephanie was now over twenty years old and still needed daily schooling in basic academics as well as learning how to manage household chores. Dr. Frostig knew of no other facility where Stephanie could reside for a limited time and learn to become independent. All other placements would be permanent care facilities. It reminded me of 1971, when we had been desperate to find a school for Stephanie until we found the Frostig Center.

Dr. Frostig's praise weighed in heavy in my decision to look at WTP as soon as possible. She explained that most of the *clients* of WTP—as they were called—had suffered brain damage at birth. These young people were able to learn how to perform rudimentary tasks, and WTP sought to prepare them for living in the community by training them in jobs they could perform adequately. Routinely. There were a few clients who had behavioral problems, but this was to be expected. "But don't worry," Dr. Frostig said, "they are not much different from the students at the Frostig Center."

I took Stephanie with me when I first visited the facility, and within a short time they accepted her. Then my adventurous daughter got herself ready for the challenge of living in a place with dozens of other young adults.

Work Training Programs was located in Chatsworth in the San Fernando Valley. It was an easy thirty-minute drive from our house, separated by the Santa Monica Mountains from the Westside where we lived. We had no friends there and were not familiar with that part of the greater Los Angeles area. When the home of WTP came into view, we saw it was a pleasant-looking two-storied building, much like a convalescent home. Only here it was filled with young faces and their lively voices. And rock music blasting from radios.

Stephanie eagerly moved in Monday morning. On the first Sunday, she and some clients in her age group were given permission to go for a walk in the quiet neighborhood. One of the boys asked Stephanie to carry his boom box, and because the boy was cute, she did. Then the boy and some of the others skipped off. She found herself alone, holding the heavy box. No one had advised her to take the address and phone number of the facility with her.

She got lost. Soon she grew tired, and the longer she walked, the heavier the radio-cassette player became. However she felt responsible and did not want to abandon it. Flushed with the summer's heat, sweaty and tired, she sat down to rest on the curb in front of a house behind a white picket fence. Flowers bloomed in profusion in the garden, and Stephanie felt (she told me later) that whoever lived there would be a nice person. Her instinct turned out to be correct. A widow and former schoolteacher had noticed her through the curtains and came out to ask her if she was lost. Yes, she confessed, I am. She did not tell her she lived in the facility of Work Training Program, but while sipping the good Samaritan's lemonade, Stephanie gave her several of the phone numbers she remembered. First she called me: I was not home. Then she called her grandmother, who was also out. She did not call her father, but called Michelle, her close friend from the Frostig Center—meanwhile a graduate from a Catholic high school—with a job and a car. She was in luck. Michybug, as we called her, was home. She jumped into her Toyota, and within a relatively short time arrived at the address in the Valley the nice lady had given her, taking one of the canyons that cut through the mountain chain from the Pacific Palisades where she lived.

Michelle was like a second daughter to me and was thoroughly familiar with our house. She even knew where I kept a spare key hidden, and she was able to let them both in. They helped themselves to ice cream and played music until I came home, surprised to find them in the den. The next day Stephanie and I went to the WTP facility and brought back the fatal boom box. I confronted the director and complained that there was not enough supervision for these kids with brain-related problems. He made light of the episode and dismissed me. I packed Stephanie's clothes and took her home.

A few months later, the house on Ridgedale Drive, home to us for more than twenty-four years, was sold. I bought a house in Santa Barbara, about ninety miles north of Los Angeles.

It was a sad parting, for Stephanie and for me when I said goodbye to the house that had sheltered us. I felt connected to it. I loved it, and the house still loved me. I said goodbye to the garden and to the by-now-very-large Jacaranda tree I planted in front of Steven's window when we first bought the house—a tree with blue blossoms. I had bought the tree for him, since we knew that would soon be his room. Since Marvin left, it showered the front lawn with an overabundance of deep blue blossoms, almost purple, as if mirroring my sadness, my *blues*. Or was the tree trying to compensate me for my sadness?

Our lives moved on, and crying over what could not be reversed was of little use. We were confident that moving to a smaller town was best for both of us. Stephanie's safety was one of the factors adding a positive weight to the equation. If she were to pass her driver's test in the future—and both she and I hoped that she would—I'd panic each time she'd come home late if we still lived in the Los Angeles area. And if Stephanie were to fail her tests, I knew the buses in the large metropolitan area would not be safe for her. One wrong bus, one missed stop, and she could end up in gangland. In Santa Barbara, the MTD bus line had a connecting hub in the center of town, and each bus returned after its route to this hub. She could not get lost.

My decision was also influenced by finances. Our big house on Ridgedale Drive was the first and only house I had called my own. Now I would have to scale down. Way down. The move to Santa Barbara, this complete change of scene, transformed my downsizing necessity into an adventure.

Chapter Twenty-Three

The Golden City

Birds fly
Flowers bloom
The sun
The moon
The night
All make me feel alive
The waves in the ocean blue
The mountaintops
And crystal skies
I love them so
—Stephanie Finell, October 1993

The sun appeared behind billowing clouds as we neared Santa Barbara on Highway 101. The Pacific to our left glittered metallic, dotted by otherworldly invaders, squatting on spidery legs in the shimmering sea; utilitarian ugliness —oil platforms. And beyond in the distance floated the Channel Islands.

My heart grew lighter as we came nearer to our new home. I opened the window of the U-Haul truck I was driving. Air rushed in, smelling of iodine-seaweed and salt, fresh and pure after the recent days of rain. Stephanie and I looked at each other at the very same time, and we both broke out in silly Cheshire-cat grins.

We turned off the freeway onto streets winding toward the hills. The street names rolled off the tongue like names of songs: Milpas, Indio Muerto, Salinas, Orizaba, reminding us of Santa Barbara's Spanish past. The whitewashed homes and their red-tiled rooftops made me feel as though we were driving somewhere in Andalusia.

I squeezed her. "Happy?" I asked.

"I love it here. I'm so glad we're leaving L.A."

"Ooops, I almost missed our turnoff," I said, swinging the truck to the right and onto our quiet cul-de-sac.

There, our new house came into view, situated on a small hill, surrounded by nature. The land—a wild mass of blue, sprinkled with dots of orange—seemed to smile at us. I thought them to be wildflowers, but they had been seeded and thoroughly watered. Statice and California poppies, still blooming now in November.

We drove up, opened our front door. *Our new home.*

"Mom, we're the first people here, no ghosts."

"Why would there be ghosts?"

"Remember? The lady who bought our old house made you go to every corner of the house and tell it goodbye. . .she said there'd be ghosts."

"Oh that. Yes. . .rather odd. She was convinced the house wouldn't want me to leave it. But. . .no more talk of the old. This house, do you love it? *We* picked it, Stephanie. No man's opinion necessary. Our taste alone."

"It's perfect. Perfect, for you and me."

And indeed, it was.

It was November 1985, and we approached our third Thanksgiving without husband and father. Mother drove up from Santa Monica for the day. I felt I should have been over my feelings of loss by now, but I was not. Thanksgiving had traditionally been the holiday dedicated to Marvin's family, and I felt sad and nostalgic. There was little joy in baking, or making my special turkey stuffing. Mother and Stephanie were appreciative, but I missed Marvin's eyes lighting up when he smelled the German apple cake coming out of the oven, and Rose's approving nod when I presented it at the table. I felt an emptiness during this holiday, and the hollow space under my ribs hurt.

We were both more cheerful when Christmas came. Our new house was less formal than the old one, and the whitewashed lath-and-plaster walls decorated with green pine garlands and lacquer-red poinsettias looked indeed like Christmas.

Soon Stephanie started classes at another branch of Work Training, Inc., but here in Santa Barbara, she lived at home and would attend classes for six hours a day, five days a week. The school was located about a fifteen-minute drive from our house. It seemed ideal.

On weekends we set out to explore our new city. The beaches, State Street, shops, movie houses, the many parks and museums, especially the butterfly collection in the Natural History Museum which Stephanie dragged me to over and over again. We also visited this museum at night, and looked at the stars through its telescope, watched the heavens in its planetarium, and when we came home and looked at the stars from our own front terrace we found harmony. In Los Angeles we had forgotten how beautiful a night sky could be.

In the spring of 1986, a family friend gave Stephanie a six-week-old German shepherd. Stephanie called her Capri, since the pup was born under the sign of Capricorn. She was a ball of fur with two pointed ears and a pink tongue sticking out, and she ran from the kennel straight into Stephanie's arms.

Capri became our protector. She grew quickly, and her fierce attack-dog look would scare some people, but anyone who took a moment to get to know her soon found her to be all play and love.

The beach became her favorite outing, where she turned into a surf dog, crashing through the waves after her stick. She rode the crest back like a surfboard made of foam, then leaped into the water to chase the stick again and ride yet another wave. We took her hiking to Paradise Road and Red Rock, where she went diving after stones in the river, and to Nojoqui Falls, where she splashed behind the curtain of water. A German shepherd? It seemed that she was more sea lion than dog.

But there were dark moments in our lives. Stephanie missed her father terribly. He and Judith, by now his wife, often spent weekends in Solvang, located twenty miles beyond Santa Barbara in the Santa Ynez Valley. It was then that Stephanie saw her father, while he passed through town. Stephanie was always in a happy mood before his visit. But he usually brought her back in less than an hour, after a brief lunch. Steff would cry and complain that the visits were too short, and why did he always have to bring *her* along. Even on the day when Marvin and Judy stayed at the nearby Biltmore, the visit was brief.

"Dad doesn't love me. Why can't he leave her there for an hour and come alone?"

"Steffi, he loves you, but he's married now. Maybe she doesn't like to be alone. He wants to make her happy."

"But this makes *me* unhappy. I told him I would like to see him alone, just once."

A few days later Stephanie felt lonely and phoned him. The machine answered. He didn't return her call.

That night Steff's eyes were red-rimmed. I wanted so much to help her, but she kept silent. I watched her scribble in her notebook, tearing pages out, crumpling them, throwing them in the trash. Later I found a poem among the scraps of paper.

FOR DAD
Today I am me, tomorrow I'll be gone.
I don't know any more.

What I feel in my heart
It's like a nightmare
And I'll never wake up
From this darkness.
But please,
I hope I shall one day,
And I hope, my Dad will wake up,
And come back. . .

—Spring 1986, Stephanie Finell

It touched me deeply, her scribbled poem, and I remembered the note she had written when we were still in Africa: *I hope, I hope, / That soon my Dad will wake up / I hope, I hope, / And come back one day.* These were similar thoughts, and I knew that Stephanie's pain had not eased off.

Not being able to help her increased my own pain. No, her dad would not come back. Had I nourished false hopes by saying I had forgiven him and that I still loved him? How could I make Stephanie understand that one can love on different levels? Yes, I did love him still, but not as one loves a husband. I loved him like a relative, as a part of my past. He was someone I had known intimately for almost half of my life. He was someone with whom I had shared my happiest moments and my saddest. But I would never want him back as a husband. I had discovered he was a terribly flawed human being. But then, who was I to judge? I would be there as a friend if he needed me. Nothing more.

I put Stephanie's poem and my thoughts aside and kissed her goodnight. Suddenly her lips quivered and tears filled her eyes.

"Stephanie, what is it?"

"It's fucked Mother, totally fucked."

"Steffi! What's wrong?"

"Dad. That's what's wrong. How can he? She's his cousin, they're. . .It's like marrying your uncle or. . .He must be crazy or something."

"I thought you and I were happy here in Santa Barbara?"

"I *am* happy. But I want my dad. He doesn't answer my calls. I was gonna swim to Anacapa this afternoon. . ."

"You. . .what?"

"When I was at the beach with the girls from Work Training? You know, Lisa? She was already dressed. . .in her sweats, waiting. It got all foggy, and I went back in the water and wanted to go and swim far out into this. . .this. . .to the island. To Anacapa. I thought, maybe I'll reach it, maybe I won't. Then he'll be sorry—"

I caught my breath, pulled her to me, and held her very tight. "Stephanie, Stephanie. Don't even think those thoughts. . .not ever again. I don't know what —" I sniffed, wiped my eyes with my sleeve. "What would I do without you?"

"Mom. . .I didn't, now, did I?"

"Hush away with these thoughts. You are very much loved. I'll always be here for you, you know that. And your daddy loves you. He shows it as much as he can. Men, well, some men, are not as demonstrative as women. I feel sorry for him."

I watched her sad expression change to a half smirk lifting the corners of her mouth, while her eyes still held tears. "Really! Mom!" She shook her head. "Somehow I can't feel sorry for him. But I do for me. I've lost my father." Then she slung her arms around me and squeezed hard. "'Nite, Mom. Love you."

I later wondered if Marvin had received Stephanie's calls. There had been an incident when she was supposed to meet him in Los Angeles. It had taken longer to retrieve my car from the repair, five miles from where he lived, than I had anticipated. I called and left a message. When I finally met Marvin at the entry to his condo, there was only half an hour's time left for them to see each other. Had he been given my message, he could have had more than an hour with his daughter. When I told him I had called and spoken to Judith and left her the message of the reason for our tardiness, he became furious, "God dammit," he said. "That woman keeps me hog tied. She never gave me the message, goddamned jealous bitch."

Stephanie and I had looked at each other, and rolled our eyes in surprise at this outburst. That is the only time I saw a glimmer of the old lion Marvin rattling the shackles in his cage. He dropped Steffi off at Ulrike's house in Beverly Hills thirty minutes later, Judith by his side, and Stephanie hopping out of the back seat.

I reminded Stephanie of that episode, and that perhaps there were more messages left on her father's machine that he never received. Steff looked at me and shook her head. "No, Dad doesn't want to call me back. He feels guilty when he's with me. He's weird."

In December 1986, after we celebrated our second Christmas with Mother in Santa Barbara, she had a severe car accident on Pacific Coast Highway. I'd begged her not to go to Malibu to visit her friend on Sunday during Christmas week. I argued there would be holiday traffic, but she was eager to see Isolde before the New Year. A station wagon emerged suddenly from a parking lot to her right, and her reflexes were too slow to avoid it. It hit her broadside, breaking her hip and her ankle. Worse than the breaking of bones, however, was that when she was coming out of the anesthesia after her hip replacement, Mother suffered a stroke. She would never be the same independent woman again.

It was early in March 1987, and Mother was staying at my house recuperating. She had been discharged from the rehab facility in Los Angeles, and I had to find a caretaker for her before she would be able to return to her apartment in Santa Monica.

I walked on the beach with Capri one morning, and Mother, impatient-ly waiting for me in my Suzuki jeep hailed a passer-by, walking on the sand. "Young man," she demanded in her German-accented voice, "Please find my daughter walking her dog. She's been gone much too long."

There were few people on the beach on this spring morning, and the young man marched off to do this old lady's bidding. He returned after a while, shook his head, no, he had not seen a woman with a dog.

My mother, not one to give up easily, sent him off again. "You must find her, young man!" she insisted. "There is hardly anyone on the beach, you can't miss her. Blonde, with this German shepherd, please, go and find my daughter. Her name is Karin. I can't stand it here any longer. . .I can't. I had a hip operation, you see? Please—"

What was he to do? Off he went again. By this time I had rounded a rocky promontory, and he did see me. He called out, "Are you Karin?"

I thought, *Who is this handsome young man who knows my name? Has Warren Beatty materialized here on the beach in Santa Barbara?* And my heart beat a little faster.

He introduced himself, "My name is Martin Dent," he said.

"Dent? I have a friend, he was my favorite English professor at UCLA. His name is Dent. Robert Dent. Are you two perhaps related?"

He smiled and shook his head. We fell in step, and while we walked back to Mother in the jeep, his accent told me he was from Britain. He told me he came from my favorite part of the island, "Wordsworth country," the Lake District. He had recently been to India, and I told him about my trip to India and La-dakh, and as we walked, we chatted of faraway places. Then he asked me about Santa Barbara.

"Do you have one of Santa Barbara's fabled gardens?" he asked.

"No, I'm afraid not," I said. "It's a rather untamed garden. I only moved here a little more than a year ago, and my house was just built and stood in a virtual wilderness when I bought it."

"I'd love to see it, if you allow me to."

"Are you a gardener?"

"No," he smiled, "I studied economics but I am more interested in unusual plants and gardens than in looking at financial data."

We stayed up late that night and talked about a million things, about nature, his interests in traveling to wild places, his ideas for my garden. He told me sto-ries about regions in Turkey and Afghanistan. He had spent time on a kibbutz in Israel and worked harvesting grapes in France during his college days. To refinance his globetrotting ways, he had harvested and even canned tomatoes in Australia. He spoke fluent French and good enough Spanish, a little Turkish and quite a bit of German, and I found him utterly intriguing. He looked like someone a Tarot card reader had prophesied to me three years ago: "A tall and slender young man will walk toward you and into your life. He is very different from you, he is a man aligned to nature, not at all sophisticated. Despite your differences, you will be compatible and find happiness with him."

I tried not to, but I fell in love with this man, years younger than myself. Yes, this was madness, but then I remembered my mother "introduced" us. Didn't she? Mother's first car accident in 1960 had brought me to her lawyer's offices, where I met Marvin Finell. From Marvin to Martin. Car accidents. The irony: I had not liked the name Marvin and often wished his name were Martin. Sometimes wishes come true.

Stephanie begged me to let her be in the advanced "Independent Living" program, that WTP Inc. had recently begun in Santa Barbara. I had heard that the Santa Barbara program was run differently from the one in Los Angeles, and I knew from the day programs that the teachers were kind. Here Stephanie had fun on supervised outings to the beach, playing volley ball and other games.

Four girls would share a two-bedroom apartment on the Mesa, a pleasant residential area in Santa Barbara. They would live by themselves, with supervision both in the morning and in the evening. Vans took the clients to and from the school Stephanie already attended. They lived close to a mini mall, where students could learn to shop independently. There were several small restaurants and fast food places in the area as well. Our house could be reached in twenty minutes by car. I hoped Stephanie would not get lost. We were asked if Stephanie took birth control pills, and, though there was no man in her life, the gynecologist here in Santa Barbara had advised me to keep her safe from an unwanted pregnancy and suggested she wear a patch.

Stephanie was enthusiastic about the program, and it seemed to me, she would live much as if she were a college student in a dorm.

She loved the varied subjects in the studies program, where she excelled in geography. Her travels had taught her quite a bit. She had high hopes of finding a job and becoming independent once she completed the program.

When I met one of her roommates though, alarm bells went off. The girl had terribly inflamed gums. Swollen and bleeding gums. I asked the young woman in charge what malady afflicted the girl. What if the girls switched toothbrushes by mistake, perhaps the girl's gum condition was contagious. She said, "Don't you worry, she's taking Dilantin, that's a very powerful anti-convulsing drug and causes this condition. It is not contagious. The poor girl is already losing some of her teeth."

I nodded. I remembered I was warned of those aftereffects when Stephanie was taking Dilantin more than twelve years ago. I wondered why the doctors had not taken this girl off that medicine and put her on Tegretol or Mebaral. Perhaps it was a question of who would pay for the more expensive drugs. I said a silent *thank you* that Stephanie had been seizure free and had not taken medicines for several years.

Aida felt no longer needed and left us to return to Guatemala.

I boarded Capri with a neighbor and went on a trip to the Southwest with Martin, where I did research for a novel in progress.

When I came back and embraced my Stephanie, I noticed an ugly red welt on her right lower arm. "What is this?" I asked the supervisor at the apartment, pointing to the scar. She shrugged and said, "Oh, it's nothing. It's from cleaning out the oven."

"Cleaning out what oven?"

"You know, the kids have to share their housework, keeping the apartment clean. And it was Stephanie's turn to clean the oven."

I looked at the welt again. About four inches long, an inch wide, shiny and dark-pinkish red. "That's how she got *that*? From the oven?"

"Well maybe it was the oven. They had put the oven cleaner in, you know it has to be set at the highest temperature, and she went in there—"

"Excuse me! You mean you let a brain-injured girl whose right arm is insensitive and partially paralyzed clean out an oven? Who supervised this? She couldn't possibly do this by herself. Where you present when this happened?"

"I,. . .no. Someone was there and they put cold water on it."

"Cold water? Didn't someone take her to the ER? There is poison in oven cleaning sprays, something had to be done!" By now I screamed, "What was done?"

Cold water. And now it had healed poorly into a huge welt. Stephanie was lucky it did not get badly infected. I packed Stephanie's belongings and took her home with me. That was the end of Work Training Program for us.

I learned that "programs" did not work for Stephanie's particular case of brain damage. I noticed, and came to believe, that those who were born healthy and had suffered brain damage at a later age, were affected with a great variety of symptoms, since their brain was affected in different parts of the cerebral cortex. The clients in places like WTP had been born with specific problems, which were easier to diagnose and classify, and their behavior in the majority of cases was easier to predict. Stephanie was not cut out to be in a program where a "one size fits all" curriculum is applied.

Stephanie faced another problem, too. What some call the invisible "illness" people with brain injuries suffer. People who did not know her well, expected more from her than she could deliver. When she was aware of her own forgetting, she would try to hide it in order not to appear "stupid." Many people saw her as smart, receptive, and able to understand and learn. This was true, but only intermittently. She could remember facts today, but maybe not tomorrow. If I wanted my daughter to be safe, I had to take care of her myself. I had to be the one to help her gain a certain amount of independence.

Chapter Twenty-Four

Special Olympics

Santa Barbara had a few distinctive neighborhoods, most of them close to the Pacific. Through WTP we had both become acquainted with the Mesa, a safe middle-class area where we rented an apartment on Rose Avenue for Stephanie, not far from where she had lived with the three other girls from WTP. It was a nice two-bedroom apartment, with a view of the sea, which she shared with a UCSB student in her late twenties. But she, too, turned out to be unreliable. Then Aida, our wonderful Aida, came back. She had missed *her* Stephanie—and I suspect her earnings in the United States as well.

Stephanie was acquainted with some of the stores by now and went grocery shopping by herself. She made lists of the foods they needed and accounted for the money she spent. She never carried more than twenty dollars with her and came home with the correct change. She also lived within walking distance of City College, where she attended special education and gym classes. There she took ballet again. Capri still lived at my house but was allowed to visit.

These months, however, were not without terrifying moments.

Stephanie had met Jesse, a polite and nice-looking young man in one of her remedial classes at City College. He walked her home. She whispered to me that they had kissed. When she asked him why he didn't work, he told her he was on disability because he was HIV positive. It was the beginning of the 1990s, and I had no idea that HIV was the precursor of AIDS and was contagious. How could I have been so ignorant? I sensed it was something serious, if a seemingly strong young man is considered disabled. I asked our gynecologist, Dr. Quijano, about this disease. He explained it to me. I was shocked. I knew that Stephanie had little self-control if she felt attracted to a boy. I needed information: was he bisexual? or did he get infected sharing needles when using drugs? Thinking about it, though, it didn't matter how he became infected. The frightening aspect of it was that he had become infectious with this incurable disease. I took her home to stay with me to cool things down for a few days, to gain time and then make a decision.

She stopped going to her classes. When I spoke to Aida, she told me the young man had left letters at their doorstep every day. Stephanie let me read them, and they were the sweetest—if illiterate—letters.

I was tortured with indecision. Yes, I knew she'd have to break up with Jesse, but how could I make her understand? I wished we could still purchase medieval chastity belts. She promised to see him as a friend only and never kiss him again. I knew I could not trust her promises. I needed her father to talk sense to her.

He was not alarmed when I told him. His sister was in town, and he had to be with her. "Come see us with Farol then. Both of you," I pleaded, "Please! Please come and talk to your daughter!"

"No. Judy and I are leaving town the day after tomorrow. Maybe Farol can visit you; she's going to spend a week in Ojai."

"Thank you for your help. You are the best father a girl could wish for," I said and slammed down the receiver.

Stephanie and I went to Ojai for a spa day. When I told Farol what had happened, her face grew red, and she set her mouth in a grim line. "How could he act like such a bastard," she said of her brother.

She spoke to Stephanie about the seriousness of this disease. "Stephanie, if you were infected you would die, a slow and horrible death. Our lovely Steffi, just think, you survived one terrible illness, but from AIDS there is no cure, no survival."

Stephanie bit her lower lip, and cried, "Jesse has HIV, not AIDS."

"HIV is the beginning of the disease, it develops into AIDS. Steffi please, listen. You can't go on seeing this boy. Promise me, promise your Mom, that you will stop seeing him, please?" I knew Stephanie. She had no concept of disease or death and neither would scare her. The only one she would listen to was her father, and he was in Never Never Land.

To resolve the situation, I sought Jesse out at City College and took him to lunch at a hamburger place nearby on the beach. He was open and naive when we spoke. I believed him when he said that they had not engaged in sex. "Jesse, I am very sorry for you and your HIV." I put my hand on his and swallowed my emotion when I continued. "But as a mother I have to put a stop to Stephanie seeing you." I wiped my nose with a tissue, and he stroked my hand with his other one and to my surprise he agreed.

"I know, I know. It's so hard. I love Stephanie so very much. I know it's for the best. I promise I'll stay away from her, but—God—will it be hard."

We never saw him or heard from him again.

I enrolled Stephanie in a class at Carpinteria High School, where after six months she earned a certificate, which enabled her to work as a volunteer in a nursery school, or in K-grade in a public school. It entailed a lot of driving, from my house to her apartment and then to Carpinteria, about fifteen miles from the Mesa and back again. Stephanie loved the curriculum and got along well with the other students. Her certificate enabled her to work as a volunteer for a few morning hours in the nursery school at a Methodist church on Cliff Drive, not far from her apartment. She felt proud and independent, walking to and from work.

To keep her occupied in the evenings and for her to make new friends, I took her to Jodi House, a local support group for head-injured people. There she met others who were born healthy, men and women who had suffered brain damage later in life caused by a variety of head traumas. Some had been injured in traffic accidents. One doctor, with the bluest eyes, had been caught in an avalanche on Mount Whitney. Another, an animal trainer, had suffered a bite on his head from a Siberian tiger. All joined in weekly discussions. Here they learned about government resources available for people with head injuries, and they took comfort that they were not alone with their distress and often sudden forgetfulness, and resulting confusion.

Stephanie enjoyed riding horses again, this time at Elaine Kay's Santa Barbara Therapeutic Riding Academy, in Toro Canyon. Elaine persuaded her to participate in the Special Olympics in Riverside, California.

It was morning, and Stephanie ground a boot heel in the earth and walked toward her horse. "Mom, I don't care if I win," she said, stroking the neck of her mount, an enormous gelding. "I just want to prove that I can keep my cool and be part of it all."

Proud of my daughter and her emotional maturity, I watched as she grabbed the mane and got a leg up. The coming event: Bareback, intermediate. She was seated, grabbing the reins. *Will she slide off?* I felt her nerves as if they were my own. Or were they? Stephanie appeared calm, while I cracked my knuckles.

She held the reins in both hands with confidence, keeping big black Satinas under control. She held the reins perfectly. Yet I wondered why she used both hands, when the instructors knew that her right hand was paralyzed. Looking closer, I noticed knots on the right rein and realized that the knots were an aid to her hand. I was glad I hadn't meddled and insisted she ride using only her left hand as when riding with Western gear. Elaine Kay, the academy's founder and instructor, knew exactly what she was doing.

Earlier, hundreds of colorful balloons had been released. I saw a hope for victory in each green, yellow, purple, or red globe drifting off into the blue of the beyond. All these balloons carried the dreams of the many young—or not so young—adult-children. The atmosphere was festive. I inhaled deeply, loving it all, especially the crisp early morning air rich with its grassy scent of alfalfa, mixed with the slightly sweet smell of hay, which was joined by the unmistakable odor of horse sweat and manure.

That morning many conflicting emotions surfaced in me, including some I had previously been unaware of. I saw Stephanie, my daughter, as one of the many disabled assembled here. This thought was still painful to me, even after all these years. But I also saw her as not belonging with the others, the majority of whom had been born with brain damage. Stephanie looked younger than her twenty-five years, but she appeared to be like any other young woman. Even so, her handicaps were still numerous—her spatial disorientation still affected her, her right hand was still paralyzed, she still suffered from short-term memory loss.

Seeing her look this happy though, I smiled. I watched her sitting high on her horse. I watched her pat his neck, leaning low and whispering into his quivering ear. She loved horses. I couldn't help but feel the irony of it—she, who had almost died from equine encephalitis, the deadly horse disease.

And watching her, I felt proud. She was so self-assured. She handled Satinas with ease. It was evident that being able to command such an animal gave her a sense of competence. Satinas obeyed the slightest flick of her hand. This was quite the opposite of real life, where Stephanie was the one who was always told what to do.

I had been a reluctant recruit for this trip and came only because I knew it would make Stephanie happy if I was there to cheer her on. On our long drive south, and then east, my thoughts were condescending toward the Special Olympics. I thought it was a forum for fun and games, mainly ineffective, making the participants and their parents feel important in a recreational sort of way. I felt the money might be spent more wisely on other programs.

Gradually, as I watched the events, I became utterly involved. The smiles on the upturned, expectant faces of participants wore away the last of my doubts. I became aware of the bodies of the riders, some sadly twisted by cerebral palsy. There were Down's syndrome riders, beaming moonfaced smiles as they grabbed the mane and mounted their horses. I wondered how the judges could be fair, when so many varying degrees of disabilities were represented. Slowly I began to realize, the Special Olympics were so much more than recreation. The Special Olympics gave the participants a sense of self-worth that life often denied them. It showed these people with intellectual disabilities that, when rightly motivated, they could not be stopped from achieving their goal.

Stephanie entered the arena. The announcer's voice boomed through the hand-held loudspeaker.

"Riders in the blue ring, turn your horses."

Stephanie responded with alertness. Again I felt a wave of pride. Her seat was just right, her back flat and straight. She held her legs well, knees pressed into the flanks of the horse, heels down, though she had no stirrups. Horse and rider walked around the ring in one direction, turned and walked in the other. Stephanie and her horse were both calm. I wondered, who is teaching whom to be so composed? Satinas, the old veteran of the polo field, or Stephanie, whose hands transmitted her calm attitude?

After a canter and a series of maneuvers came the last command: "Walk your horses and come to a halt facing the judges!"

Stephanie turned, walked, and stopped. Seconds ticked away. My heart pounded. Satinas shook his head; Steff patted him and then resumed her stance, reins in each of her hands. The name of the fifth place winner was announced. A young man. He left the arena with a wide grin. The fourth. The third, the bronze medal. Now they announced the silver medal. My heart pulsed a loud thump in my throat. Sounds were a blur, and then:

"The first prize, the gold medal, goes to number sixty—"

That's Stephanie's number! An unbelievable feeling rushed through me, I strained to hear the rest of the announcer's sentence, "Stephanie Finell, of Santa Barbara!"

"Yippee!" I screamed, throwing my straw hat into the air. I wiped my cheeks. Looking at Stephanie, I saw that she too was weeping.

Stephanie bent low over Satinas's head as the judge hung the gold medal around her neck. I watched her wiping her eyes with the back of her hand. The judge asked Stephanie in a quiet voice I could barely hear, "Why are you crying?"

She answered through sniffles, "Because I've never won anything." Her voice sounded muffled as she continued, "I've never achieved anything before now."

My God! That's it. Suddenly I understood. I understood with my heart. I didn't only theorize with my mind. How could I have been so dumb? Yes, that is the purpose of the Special Olympics, to instill a sense of accomplishment in the participants.

In that one moment, could winning the "real" Olympic gold be any more exciting? I glanced at her as she tried to dry her eyes while holding on to the reins. Trumpets were blaring, announcing the next scheduled event. Stephanie turned her horse and exited the arena, her face lit by happiness, while the gold medal on her chest caught a beam of sunlight, reflecting in her eyes.

Chapter Twenty-Five

Two Weddings, Three Funerals

Summer 1991

"Mom, I met the cutest guy today!" Stephanie announced, bouncing past me into the house. "A blond surfer-boy!"

Later I met the young man with the sun-streaked hair, bronzed skin, and luminous brown-green eyes.

Loren had spent the last few months in Hawaii visiting his stepbrother and, shortly after his return to Santa Barbara, attended a Jodi House meeting. That is where they met. Loren Breck, now twenty-seven years old, was nineteen when he rode his motorcycle without a helmet on New Year's Eve, crashed it into a pole, and suffered a severe head injury. It was an area near the beach with not many motorists, and he was not seen by any one for hours. Medical help and intervention was delayed for many precious hours, complicating the injury.

Both Stephanie and Loren had felt true loneliness. And now their meeting seemed providential. They were a sweet couple and appeared to be very much in love. I soon shared in their happiness. A month or so later, Loren gave her a ring encrusted with small diamonds and rubies, a ring he could barely afford. Stephanie radiated joy, and she kept holding up her hand, catching the sparkle of sunlight in the stones.

Loren's parents liked Stephanie; I in turn liked Loren, as did Marvin when he met him.

"What's not to like?" one of my friends said laconically of Loren.

He was good-looking, had a muscular body, was polite and knew his manners, and seemed to adore Stephanie. She was faster than he was in physical activities, and he had a few problems with walking, as a result from his particular brain injury. She would easily get lost in town, whereas he knew the city and the streets well. Sadly for him, when he walked down Santa Barbara's main street, State Street, especially later in the afternoon by himself, the police often stopped him thinking he was drunk. His gait at times was unsteady. He had no driver's license but an ID card, and luckily he was very good natured. He smiled and tried to explain why he walked "funny," as he called it, and the police understood. But I heard of other brain injured men who were short-tempered and would become aggressive with the police, and this led to a whole other set of problems. Loren was a happy-go-lucky guy. After he was back in Santa Barbara for a while, several men in the police force got to know him and said hello, when they saw him.

The months following their engagement were filled with the euphoria of planning their wedding, choosing china, glassware, furniture, and Stephanie's trousseau.

The wedding took place on May 2, 1992.

It was to be an informal affair, akin to a Mediterranean country wedding on a sunny California day. Approximately sixty-five guests were invited. The mountains behind our house wore springtime green. The flowers in the garden were blooming in a blaze of color from yellow to fiery orange to the deep magenta of the bougainvillea. The blades of grass reflected the sun, creating a shimmering lawn.

Loren's family and his parents' friends were numerous, and to me it felt a bit odd to greet so many unfamiliar faces. When our friends arrived, each took a seat on the left side of the aisle on the fold-up wooden rental chairs. Mother seemed very happy to see her Stephanie marrying Loren, and the smile did not leave her face all afternoon. Aida looked like a caring aunt, wearing a silken dress of black and mauve she had bought for the occasion and sporting an orchid corsage, as did my mother—compliments of the florist.

Steven had arrived from St. Louis with Beth and their two sons, Jared and Christopher. They immediately took off their dark jackets and were playing hide and seek, rustling the bushes and leaping boulders in the upper garden. This was the extent of our small family assembled here in Santa Barbara.

Then there was the bridal party, the men in tuxedos, but for (I could not believe my eyes) the father of the bride who appeared in a light beige tropical suit. I felt my face flush with anger. How could he have forgotten? I had told him—and also Judith to remind him—that the others would be wearing tuxedos. Please, see to it that he didn't have his at the cleaners. "Yes, yes, yes, don't worry, I'll wear my penguin suit," he'd said.

Allan was the best man. I don't remember why he was chosen to be the best man, but Loren's friends from childhood and high school had drifted away after his accident. His brother was married, and we had to pick a young unmarried man to accompany the young unmarried bridesmaid. Allan was Martin's friend from his wandering years in Europe and Asia, and with whom he had a long history of meeting, each time coincidentally, in the remotest of places of Greece or Turkey. As it turned out, they met again when Allan ended up here, earning his PhD in art history at the University of California at Santa Barbara. We'd seen a lot of him during the previous year or two, and I felt as if he were family. Allan became part of our small group of like minds here in town. Now he was part of the bridal party, escorting the bridesmaid—Loren's cousin and the minister's daughter, the beauteous, serious Siri.

Loren's mother, Susan, looked like the beauty queen she had once been. A few years older now, she wore the passing years well. Her chestnut brown hair was full and naturally wavy. She wore it swept up in a chignon, but strands had come lose and curled around her face in wisps. Her selection of a suit of raw silk in a soft shade of orchid was a perfect choice for the mother of the groom. She would have been the belle of the ball, were it not for the focal point, Stephanie, the radiant bride and now Susan's new daughter-in-law.

Pete, Loren's stepfather, was six foot three with a shock of silver hair and presented the picture of a debonair diplomat. He had been a dealer in antiques but, at this time, had acquired a franchise store of fine California-made chocolates. He was properly attired in a dark suit with a subtle pinstripe, and again I cringed when I looked at Marvin in his light beige suit. Then I forced my thoughts not to dwell on it.

But it bothered me for several reasons.

He knew it was important to Stephanie that everything at her wedding would go as planned. Stephanie had dreamt of a traditional white wedding with traditional music and all the rest that goes with it. Marvin was going to walk his daughter down the aisle, and he had to look like the father of the bride. Was this forgetfulness, or was it a certain disdain for what, to Stephanie, was an important and solemn occasion? Was it another example of disregard that he had shown at other times?

I recalled how he had chosen to go out of town during Stephanie's high school graduation. He knew it meant a great deal to Steffi, but he had called her graduation, "a Mickey Mouse kind of affair." Even if that diploma was not certified from her school district's high school, it meant a lot to Stephanie. The pinch in my heart was there again, this pain, that her own father considered her to be of inconsequence—on the day that was meant to be the happiest in her life. He paid for half the wedding. That was important to him. Expenses. To him she was "damaged," because of her brain injury, and I hated him for it. I only hoped that Stephanie, cocooned in her cloud of euphoria, would not notice.

This day was the first time that Judith had entered my property. We all took our seats, and I was chagrinned when she came to sit close to me during the ceremony. She kept raising her arms and rattling the heavy gold bracelets— *Were they Cartier? Obviously new and expensive.* It appeared as if she tried to get others' attention with her baubles, and I found the jangling difficult to ignore. She wore a tasteful, Chanel-type knit suit in wool, warm and wintry, the opposite of Marvin's Florida attire. How could she have let him wear that suit? Was this her doing, to show this wedding didn't matter?

It was silly of me to be so annoyed with both of them on my daughter's wedding day. But the snake of past anger with its poison of betrayal and jealousy had awakened and now crept up within me. For a moment, I tasted its bitter gall. I almost arose from my chair to sit next to Aida. (I would have sat next to Mother, but she was parked in her wheelchair in the back of the rental chairs.)

Then I took a few deep yoga breaths. I told myself to think of my good fortune. I saw Martin escorting the late arrivals to their seats. I looked over at Stephanie. Always Stephanie. She looked so beautiful in her wedding gown and the corona of flowers with her veil half-covering, half-revealing her face.

And there stood Loren, handsome in his tuxedo, the sun glinting in his brown-blond hair. He looked flushed with excitement. A few steps in back of him stood the best man, Allan, and Siri, the maid of honor.

I brought myself under control.

I will always remember how much Stephanie looked like Cinderella at the ball. Her white taffeta dress billowed out over its petticoat. Years ago, when she was in a coma in an oxygen tent, she had looked like another fairytale figure—Snow White, in her glass coffin. I felt my eyes filling with tears again, while at the same time feeling intensely grateful for her present health and grace as she took her father's arm to walk down the aisle. The joyous strains of "Here Comes the Bride" were played by a classical trio on our front terrace. Her white dress swooshed over the white carpet laid between the chairs leading to the arch. She almost danced at the arm of her father toward the white blossomed arch.

Here, Dr. Robert Wennberg, the officiating Presbyterian minister (Susan's brother), and Loren, the handsome groom, awaited father and daughter. But a few steps before Stephanie reached the arch, Capri walked straight across her train. I remember Steff's impish smile, when she paused for a moment, then walked on—unaware of the large brown paw prints on her white train, her hand still resting on her father's arm, calm and poised.

Dr. Wennberg spoke to the young couple in a tone of deep seriousness. They would have to be strong for each other, he said. They must surmount many obstacles in life due to their brain injuries. He hoped that the extended families would be there to help Loren and Stephanie with good advice, he said, directing his eyes from the young couple to the assembled relatives and friends. He added, that in some instances, more active help might be needed. I felt reassured by his words. Our own family was small. It was a comfort to me that Loren had so many relatives living in Santa Barbara.

After Loren and Stephanie had taken their vows, and the groom kissed the bride, they slowly turned to walk between the rows of seats accompanied by the bravos and air-kisses blown by friends. The trio now played Mendelssohn's "Wedding March" from *A Midsummer Night's Dream,* and when the rhythm picked up, Stephanie's feet followed. Loren had a bit of trouble keeping pace with her. The music sounded triumphant when they returned to Martin and me, and—to a surprise: Uncle Bud Seretean had arrived at the last minute with Cousin Tracy. Stephanie's face beamed when he bent to kiss her.

As the Moët Chandon corks popped, the brash sound of a trumpet heralded a change of beat. The classical trio made way for a group of Mariachis, appearing with their varied instruments, as if accompanying the popping champagne corks.

The sixty or so wedding guests followed the Mariachis to the back of the house where the buffet was laid with its feast of delicacies: there was hot tri-tip, enchiladas, breast of chicken, cold cuts of ham and sliced beef, and Stephanie's and my favorite, poached salmon with capers on a bed of parsley. The guests found their places at large round tables with tablecloths of a deep pink, napkins of a lighter shade, and flower arrangements of a mix of hothouse and wild flowers. Stephanie had specifically asked for California's orange poppies—but they would wilt too quickly and Iceland poppies of that same hue were substituted. The orange color added spice to the varied pink shades of roses, all intermixed with white daisies and delicate baby's breath. All of this was Stephanie's idea. She remembered some of the lessons from the class in flower arranging she had taken in Santa Monica City College.

Stephanie danced the first dance with her father. Her eyes sought only his face. She glowed when he held her and swirled her as of old. Loren's turn came next. Loren's dancing was a bit stiff, but to me the two looked just like any happy young couple.

Then again, I felt on edge because of Judith. Wherever I went to mingle with our guests, I could hear those bracelets jangling. I told myself over and over not to let *her* spoil my happiness on this wonderful day. But it annoyed me when she went over to the caterer to whisper in her ear—so everyone else could hear—that she was going to have an important party with some very important guests at her condo in Beverly Hills. Would the caterer consider catering the same menu there? I wondered why she would want to imitate my daughter's wedding buffet. There were excellent caterers in Los Angeles. Why would she want me and others to know that she had *very important guests*?

When she danced with Marvin, she danced so suffocatingly close that the poor man—normally a fine dancer, light on his feet and matching the best dancers' fancy steps—could hardly move. He could only shuffle. Every so often she cast a triumphant glance at me.

After the meal and the cake ceremony (no, Stephanie did not want any cake in her face), after the dancing and after Marvin and my nemesis had left, the Mariachis sounded the last trumpet's hurrah. Guenther, our Austrian neighbor volunteered to drive the newlyweds to the Fess Parker Hotel. It was located by the seashore, and they were going to spend their wedding night there, a wedding gift from Loren's brother, David. I saw Stephanie and Loren get into

Guenther's gold-colored Mercedes convertible, with Stephanie squishing her big skirt inside and climbing onto a high pile of cushions in the back seat of the open car. Guenther took the longer route down State Street—busy on this late Saturday afternoon with shoppers but also with very slow traffic and, luckily, no cops. They could have gotten into trouble not wearing seatbelts. Stephanie felt like a princess, seated so high, waving to pedestrians as they blew her kisses and waved back.

Most, but for one young man who shouted: "Suckers!"

Martin and I, plus Allan and Siri, followed in our car, and we were slightly amused by the entire spectacle.

A few days after the wedding we were shown an enchanting cottage hidden within an overgrown "English" garden in the San Roque part of Santa Barbara, a ten-minute drive from my house. The house was located on Paseo Tranquillo, appropriately named "Tranquil Street," to fit with the quiet neighborhood. It was ideal for the newlyweds. When Loren and Stephanie saw the house they were enthusiastic. Loren liked plants and gardening and told me he would be happy to take care of the pruning of bushes and mowing the small lawn. He immediately had plans for planting flowers and making a vegetable garden in the rear of the house. Stephanie looked at him in admiration, "You can do all that Loren?" He smiled his typical Loren smile, lips closed and spread from ear to ear, his hazel eyes twinkling. "But of course. Ask my Mom, I help them with the garden all the time."

I made an offer on the house. I knew I would have to be able to finalize this purchase. (A trust fund, from Marvin's parents, made this possible.)

Buying a house had become a necessity, since Aida still had to live with Stephanie and Loren to help them in their daily routine. The lease for Stephanie's apartment specified that only two adults were to live in the apartment. I had looked for a place to rent for them and found it next to impossible to rent anything, apartment or house for a young couple afflicted with handicaps, unless the rental was tied to a government program, such as Section 8 for which Loren, but not Stephanie, qualified. There were so many government stipulations. Some were age-related, how old a person was when the injury occurred (Loren was nineteen, only half a year above the cut-off date of eighteen). And other situations played a role. Everything that is logical in our everyday world becomes an obstacle course if it involves people with handicaps or head injuries.

While the house was in escrow, Stephanie, Loren, Martin, and I went to Hawaii, on *their* honeymoon.

We were needed as overseers, since neither Stephanie nor Loren drove a car. Nor would they be able to handle bills, tips, and all the mundane things we—as Stephanie would say, "normal" people—took for granted.

I had been to Kauai before and had stayed in a small hotel with apartment-like accommodations by the beach. To give the honeymooners some privacy, Martin and I stayed in one of those condos, while they stayed at one of the elegant old Hawaiian hotels nearby. There they had room service breakfasts and some fancy evening meals by themselves, watching Hawaiian floorshows by candlelight. I went over to help Stephanie select her outfits and her bathing suits, hang her wet bathing suits up properly to dry, and pick up her strewn-about clothes. The four of us explored the island in our rental car. We hiked in Waimea Canyon and along the treacherous path of the Kalalau Trail on the steep Na Pali coast, where we bathed beneath rushing waterfalls—waterfalls of surprisingly ice-cold mountain water, making us shiver until the Hawaiian sun warmed us again.

My mind's eye sees them still, hugging and kissing, their tanned bodies wet and glistening, sleek as sea creatures, snorkeling above the coral reef on Kee Beach, swimming among the many colored fish.

Happiness and sadness came in peaks and hollows, like waves in the sea. There were weddings, and there were funerals in 1992.

Stephanie's friend Hugi married in July, but shortly after this joyous wedding, Stephanie's Aunt Farol died of bone cancer. Before her death, she spoke of being grateful to God for her last months of life. She had realized that material possessions meant little, that what mattered was loving others and acting accordingly. Then, surrounded by those she loved, she slipped into unconsciousness never to awaken again.

A short month later Marvin's mother, Stephanie's Gammy, died. Stephanie had not seen her Gammy for several years. She had lived in a home for Alzheimer's patients. Her death came as a release for her.

In early December, Stephanie and I traveled to Guadalajara. Loren at that time opted to visit his brother who had moved to Idaho. Again we felt the balm of being in the midst of Carmen and Alonso's large family. We combined this visit with a week in Rio Caliente, a health spa nearby, where we took advantage of the healing mineral waters. We'd visited the spa before and always met interesting guests. This time we made friends with a clairvoyant. She warned me, "Karin, there is much unfinished business between your mother and you. Try to make amends once you get back home. You don't have much time."

We arrived in Santa Barbara late on December 17, with a great deal to prepare before Christmas. It was up to me to decorate our two houses. This was Stephanie's first holiday in her own home, and Stephanie, ever the enthusiastic one, had invited over thirty members of Loren's family (by way of her mother-in-law, Susan) for an open house on Christmas Eve. After our return home, I visited Mother in her convalescent home every day. But never for long. And we never talked at length about our past history.

Then on December 23, Mother called me at 10:30 a.m. "Where am I going to spend Christmas Eve?" she asked.

"I'll pick you up around five and take you to Stephanie's house. You'll meet many of Loren's family that night."

"I can't get into her house with my wheelchair," she said.

"Martin will make a little ramp for you with boards. You're going to be fine."

"No. No. I want to go to your house."

"We'll be at my house on Christmas Day, Mother."

"Where will I be on Christmas Eve?"

"I told you, I'll take you to Stephanie's house where—"

"But on Christmas Day? Where will I be on Christmas Eve?'

"Mother, let's not go around in circles. You will be with all of us both days. I'll pick you up early tomorrow evening for the party at—"

"I want to know where—" She'd interrupted me again. Then she was silent for a moment, "Oh, I forgot. Aren't you coming over to see me tonight?"

"I wasn't going to. I have so many errands to run, two Christmas trees still to decorate—"

"You mean you're not going to see your old mother today? You come! I want to see you."

"Mutti, I'll stop by, but it won't be for long. I have to go now." I heard her voice rumbling but not forming words.

I said, "Sorry. I have to hang up. I'll see you in the afternoon. Have to go. Bye."

I waited for a brief acknowledgment, then I hung up. Later I wondered if I should have waited a minute longer? An hour later came the phone call. Mother had died. Suddenly. And I had ended our phone call on an exasperated note. In fact I had hung up on her. There had been no time to make amends. And she, who loved Christmas so very much, died before this year's holidays were to begin.

Martin and I were on our way to the nursing home minutes after the call. We passed Stephanie's house and stopped to let her know. She and Loren wanted to come along, and I cut white roses in their garden to take to Mother.

How did I remember to take the CD player along, and the white candles? Gregorian Chants were playing, and the white candles, which I had placed next to Mother's bed, gave off a soft glowing light. I placed the white roses below her hands. We surrounded Mother with music and prayers. Stephanie was very tender with her grandmother. She stroked her hands, her hair, and told her how much she loved her.

The funeral director came by. Stephanie rolled her eyes, noting like me the false tone in his rehearsed solemnity.

Later, in the funeral home, Mother looked peaceful. The beauty of her hands, now relaxed, startled me—they belied the fact that she had been a weaver, and a painter, and had never worn gloves while doing any kind of work. I kissed those hands and remembered the times when I was a child and had clung to them, when they had held mine so protectively.

I hoped that Stephanie would cancel her open house on Christmas Eve, but to please Loren she did not. Stephanie and I didn't feel like celebrating, but the conveyor belt of strangers' faces moving in circles around us momentarily numbed our sadness. Amid all this, Martin picked up Steven from the airport. Stephanie wept on her brother's broad, familiar shoulder. Brother and sister shared their loss.

We all went to the mortuary on Christmas Day. By now Mother wore a white satin robe I'd bought the day before. The man standing behind me in line at the lingerie counter heard me say to the salesclerk that the robe was for my mother. He said, "What an elegant gown, bet your mom's going to like it."

"Maybe," I smiled a rueful smile, "if she could see it. She died yesterday. This is for the funeral home."

"I'm so sorry," he stuttered, looking mortified, but I assured him I did not mind his remark. How could he have known? "She liked elegant clothes. She would have liked to hear your opinion."

Mother looked regal in her robe. When I touched her hands, they felt very cold. So unnatural. My mother, cold and removed and far away. I no longer could ask any of the many questions that remained unanswered. She was no more. Of late, we had loved too little; we had talked too little. Regrets, ah yes, I had them. I loved her deeply, despite our past problems. Deeply, as did Steven, as did Stephanie.

Bereaved. Finally I understood the meaning of this Victorian-sounding word. One felt bereft. Something had been taken away, stolen. Something was gone.

Forever gone.

Chapter Twenty-Six

Changes

The residents of Santa Barbara are fortunate to have excellent adult education classes associated with the local city college. Stephanie expressed an interest in some of the authors' lecture programs. I took her along to several and later found two short essays she had written in February 1993.

The Nature of Being Handicapped
by Stephanie Finell Breck

Today I met Jonathan Winters at a class at City College. He inspired me to write. I was actually shy to meet a man of his stature. He is feeling, he is witty, he is everything. And he is a Scorpio, like me!

This is my story: I was a very young girl of seven, when I was in Mexico. I had an illness called encephalitis caused by mosquito bites. It just blows my mind that this tiny insect can cause such a terrible illness. Later I was in the hospital for six weeks, in a coma. The doctor said to my parents, she will not walk or talk for the rest of her life. But I didn't believe that, neither did my parents. I was taken out of my regular school, El Rodeo, and put into a special school called the Marianne Frostig Center, and that great lady was going to retire at that time.

I feel better knowing that I had a problem, than if I were without it. There are many things I see and experience that I would be too busy to see and feel otherwise. I also don't have to worry about taxes and all of the other things that people are worrying about.

The best time is being alone, writing.

I met my husband at a place for the head injured, called Jodi House, named after a girl who died after having had a double or triple encephalitis and coma, caused by a car accident. Sadly she died.

I wish I could talk out in public about what people should know about head injuries. Maybe one given day I can talk to people about it. Most people don't really know and understand. There is the case of Dr. Schwimmer with the bluest

199

eyes, he is always smiling and he is really sweet, yet he is quadriplegic and one can hardly understand his talk.

Dr. Schwimmer is an older gentleman and I do mean *gentle man*. He had a severe head injury through an avalanche that killed his fiancée.

I feel so sorry for him, but every sad event has a meaning, I hope.

The Little Girl Inside of Me.

I was a happy little girl growing up. Everyone loved me, and everything I got for free. Happiness all around me. I found the love I got from my family, I found it on my Daddy's lap—I was his little girl.

For a while Stephanie and Loren were happy. Aida lived with them, since neither of them was able to cook or keep house. They kept attending the Jodi House meetings, which provided them with contacts and a degree of a social life. Sundays they walked several blocks to a nearby Presbyterian church. They liked going to the Museum of Natural History, also within walking distance from their home, and since they had a membership they went there often. Stephanie visited her favorite butterflies exhibit, while Loren was intrigued by the Chumash Indian artifacts. Both liked it when I took them to Mass at the Santa Barbara Mission. Both of them enjoyed music, and I bought season tickets for them to the Civic Light Opera.

Stephanie kept up with her horse riding, and during the winter months she began to ski. This also took place under the auspices of the Special Olympics and was organized by the Santa Barbara Parks & Recreation Department. They skied at Big Bear Mountain, which is the highest peak in the San Bernardino mountain chain, rising east of the Los Angeles basin. It is a four-hour drive from Santa Barbara.

I went with Stephanie a few times and was amazed how naturally she took to skiing. This, too, she must have inherited from my mother. She zoomed down the slope without poles (the method used for some handicapped beginning skiers), careening and slaloming gracefully.

On one occasion she fell into my arms at the bottom of the run, her face flushed and glowing, excitement in her eyes, "Oh, Mom! It's so great. . . woof. . .I'm out of breath. . .such a feeling. Like flying. . .try it! Really Mom, it's great."

"I'm a bit chicken. Also, I want to stay here and watch you. I'm proud of you. You don't know how much."

We stood by the lift, surrounded by a group of amputee skiers (using so-called outriggers in lieu of the missing leg). They were part of another group of disabled skiers who were in an adaptive skiing program. The group listened intently as one of the instructors—herself an amputee and one of the world's top-rated disabled female skiers—pointed out the intricacies of "one-legged" skiing. (I found the tiny skis attached to the end of their poles intriguing.)

We all watched wide-eyed as a two-legged skier shot down the hill at full speed. The man's skis crossed, spraying snow, and he flew through the air while one pole described a silver arc against the blue canvas of sky. Then followed his airborne goggles, chased by his green woolly hat. All had taken flight. He landed in a most ungraceful spill, a few feet from us. The amputees waited patiently for the man to collect his paraphernalia so they could go on with their lesson.

Then one of the group wryly remarked, "Well, that's what happens if you have two skis."

Stephanie added her little bit of wisdom, "And two poles!"

Here Stephanie found humor and camaraderie. I wished there would be more support for programs that enable the physically impaired to experience this type of activity.

One member of our group was a woman paraplegic in her late twenties who was injured by an auto accident. She skied sitting on a sled-like affair, a *sitzski*. When she landed near us after coming down the mountain, Stephanie asked, "Isn't it great?"

A smile lit the woman's fresh face, her skin aglow from sun and air, and she laughed. "Oh yeah, I love the wind in my face, the feeling of speed. Of freedom, wow! Only the mountain can do that for me."

I marveled at the possibilities for the blind, the deaf, cerebral palsy sufferers, persons with spinal-cord injuries, or polio victims. For all these people with a large variety of physical handicaps, the glorious feel of flying down a mountain on powdery white snow could become a realizable dream.

Yet I never met other parents involved in the skiing activity, perhaps because the skiers were mainly an older age group. They differed from the horse therapy group, in that most had experienced physical injuries after they were adults. Among the skiers, only Loren and Stephanie suffered from head trauma. In the horse therapy group, most of the riders were handicapped and learning impaired since birth.

Sometimes I asked myself whether it would be worse for a parent to have a child with birth defects, knowing from the outset that the child will be handicapped for life. Or was it worse to give birth to a child who starts out healthy and then suddenly suffers a dreadful event when fate snatches away the child's potential—and with it, all of the expectations the parents had for this child?

Stephanie had come along an arduous path and regained much. This might give hope to other parents—that with love and understanding, and their working with their child, the child may recover some of what was lost. I often did not feel up to the task, but I knew I must not accept defeat. The child will probably not reach the level of wholeness as before the illness or accident, but there is always the possibility that much can be brought back.

Stephanie's cold-reddened face in the doorway of the cafeteria jolted me back to the *now* when she cried out, "Hi, Mom, I'm hungry like a bear. May I have a hamburger? May I, please?"

Spring 1994

Once again Stephanie was in Big Bear, skiing under the auspices of Special Olympics. Martin and I were in Santa Fe. Early one morning I received a telephone call. An agitated woman's voice said, "Your daughter had a severe seizure while up here on—"

"Stephanie? On the slope? Did she hurt herself?"

"No, luckily she was sitting down, having lunch. But the seizure was severe. We had to take her to the hospital. It took a long time to calm her. The doctors are confident she can return with us to Santa Barbara tomorrow. Please, try and come home at once."

Martin and I took turns at the wheel and drove west, trying to outrun the course of the sun.

Stephanie had not had a seizure since 1979. That was almost fifteen years ago. Again we began our visits to doctors. She had another EEG. Since those severe seizures in Florida, Stephanie's EEGs never showed an abnormality. Now Stephanie was again put on medication.

Another severe seizure followed a few weeks later. We were driving to her polling place to vote in the municipal elections. I wanted her to be independent, to go into the booth alone, and mark her ballot. She said she was scared of forgetting what to do and marking the wrong box for the wrong candidate. A few blocks from my house she began to shake. We were in my small Suzuki jeep, which lacked the space for Stephanie to lean against a support or to lie down. After trying to calm her, I swung into a U-turn and took her back to the house. I called out for Martin. He was planting a tree in the garden. I was lucky that he could help carry Stephanie—by now limp and unconscious—into the house. I put her to bed in her former bedroom. Much like an earthquake, the seizure passed, and there were no aftershocks.

Besides the fear of seizures, there was always the terrible dread that Stephanie's mind would suddenly blank out. This is the curse of the head injured, this inconsistent short-term memory loss. Suddenly she wouldn't recognize where she was, or where she had intended to go, and had forgotten what she'd planned to do.

This type of memory loss affected many of her activities, the ability to cook, for instance, or to follow a recipe. One moment she would look at a cookbook, in the next moment she didn't remember where she'd placed the book. Or where she'd put the salt, the pepper. Even simple tasks that the Down's syndrome clients of our local Alpha Center were able to master in their cooking class at City College, Stephanie could not perform.

In theory, as during a lesson with an occupational therapist, Stephanie performed her tasks well. But later? Maybe yes. Maybe no. There was real danger in this forgetting. What if she left the gas on while a newspaper lay on the stove near the flame?

One of my greatest worries was her getting lost, wandering the streets. Several times when she was on her way to the bus, or walked the few blocks to the market, she wound up walking for miles and miles in the opposite direction.

School began in the fall, and Stephanie's certificate from Carpinteria High School came in handy. She found an opportunity to work as a volunteer—or, as she declared, "a helper" to the teacher—at Peabody Charter School, a scant four blocks from her house. After a few weeks of daily accompanied walks to and from her job, Stephanie found her way. But then, leaving the school grounds by herself, she was confronted with several streets that converged at Peabody. The choices confused her. Several times she took the wrong street and walked for hours. She was too embarrassed to ask for directions since she didn't want anyone to know she had a problem. Stephanie would rather wander the streets and get blisters than ask for help. Sometimes her exhaustion would be apparent to perfect strangers, and a kind soul would offer her a ride. Several times I nearly went crazy with worry, knowing she was lost. Then the doorbell rang and there stood Stephanie, accompanied by a police officer or a kindly woman who brought her home. Apparently she never accepted a ride from a strange man. She always gave them the address to my house, perhaps because it was our first home in Santa Barbara.

At school, Stephanie pretended to know more than she actually did. When the teacher sent her to take one of the little girls to the toilet, Steffi confessed to me, that she had no idea where the toilet was. But she told the little girl, "Hey, Susie, you know where the bathroom is. You're a big girl. You show me how smart you are." And Susie would proudly take Stephanie by the hand and lead the way. No one was ever the wiser.

Pat Morales, the principal at Peabody, was delighted to have Stephanie's help in the crowded kindergarten classroom. Stephanie's Spanish proved a bonus. She conversed with the many Latino children, recent immigrants, and could help them since their English was limited. The little ones loved her; they sensed that she truly cared for them when she focused on their needs. Stephanie wrote:

> When I was working with my kids, I was making play-dough faces, molding it into different shapes. With *both* my hands. I made paintings too. One little kid drew me a picture of his parents. When they (the children) get to know me, they like me. If one gets hurt, I'm always there for them.

And she was.

When the little ones fell and skinned their knees, she cradled them in her arms and sang them a singsong *Sana, sana, colita de rana, si no sanas hoy, sanas mañana*. She translated this to the little Anglo tykes with, "Heal, heal, tail of the frog, if you don't heal today, then you heal tomorrow."

With the children, Stephanie herself could act like a child again, and they loved her for it.

Later she wrote, *I want to have one child in my life to call my own.*

We had discussed this, and I, who would want nothing more than to have a grandchild through her, tried to curb her desire and insisted she get another birth-control arm patch.

In the beginning of her marriage, I too nourished the hope that one day Stephanie would have a child. A grandchild I could spoil, maybe a little girl who would look like her. How wonderful it would be to have a link from those who went before, through me, through Stephanie, to the future. I was as sad as she was when I realized, this could never be. And I was disappointed. Neither Stephanie nor Loren became more independent, but strangely, in this marriage, Loren lost some of his earlier self-reliance.

I had hoped that Loren would work for his mother and stepfather in the chocolate store on State Street. Loren could certainly package candies, and he could wrap them. He could help with stacking supplies, with sweeping the store. But government regulations made this plan difficult. Every penny he would earn in order to feel a bit more independent would be deducted from the small stipend he received from the government as a person with a disability. This forced Loren to stay home. To keep busy, he did some gardening, cut the hedges and watered the plants, but the plans for a vegetable garden were soon abandoned. He devoted much of his time making bead necklaces and painting small canvases of seascapes, incorporating sand from the beach and shells he had found. I admired his imagination, but again, if he were to sell them on Santa Barbara's Sunday's Crafts market on the boardwalk , he would need a license, and each penny he earned would be deducted from his monthly stipend.

Stephanie was not happy with Loren in several respects. He showed no initiative to volunteer to speak at schools about the hazards of riding a motorcycle without a helmet, which he had promised Stephanie and his parents he would do, or volunteer at the candy store, but most of the days when she came home from her job, she found him sitting on the front step smoking and drinking coffee. She had hoped to be fulfilled in a marriage, but it was not to be. Loren's mother, who really liked Stephanie, talked with her, then with Loren, and then with me. Susan wondered what we, as mothers, could do. I believed the problem had to do with brain damage and could not be solved by two caring mothers.

Still, Stephanie kept talking about having a baby. Potential scenarios frightened me. Stephanie's health and the possibility she might have seizures during her pregnancy or while giving birth were only part of it. I considered her short-term memory loss. She might place a baby into unsafe situations. When the child grew older and started high school, would I be able to help with the homework? Would I even be alive? And how would this child feel about his or her brain-damaged parents?

No, I kept shaking my head at Stephanie, trying to reason with her. It would be highly irresponsible to bring a child into the home of *two* brain-injured parents.

After Stephanie realized she could not have a child with Loren, her attitude toward him changed. He was a sweet-natured young man, but even under the best of circumstances, the day-to-day living with another head-injured person proved difficult for them. They both had problems and needs, and sometimes these could not be reconciled. Their marriage lasted two years. Then they decided to part as friends and for each to go their separate ways.

It was Sunday, May 8, 1994, at the Oaks in Ojai. It was mother and daughter week. Stephanie had a seizure on our first evening there. She babbled as if speaking in tongues, threw her arms around me, picked up her feet, and hung heavy on my neck. I let her fall onto the bed. She appeared to be out of body, acting like a somnambulist. Slowly, slowly she returned to consciousness, but she did not recognize where she was.

"We're at the Oaks, Stephanie, don't you remember?"

"What's the Oaks? Where am I?"

"The Oaks in Ojai. Sheila Cluff's place, the pretty blonde lady who is always so nice to you. Come on Steff! You remember Sheila!"

"What are we doing here? Why are we here?"

"We're here to lose weight, to exercise—" My voice trailed off to nothing. I realized Stephanie did not comprehend a single thing I was saying.

Could this seizure episode be connected to what Stephanie felt about her brother? I knew how much Stephanie worried about Steven. He was going through a very troublesome period because he and Beth were heading toward a divorce. A new man had entered Beth's life, and Steven was burning up with jealousy, frustration, and rage. I had reason to worry terribly about him. After he harangued me with telephone calls, Stephanie witnessed my sobbing into my pillow. All of this affected her. I had long suspected that there was a connection. Stress in our lives brought on seizures. Excitement often had the same effect. By the end of our Ojai week, however, life in St. Louis had normalized for Steven. There were no more seizures for Stephanie. The one-pill-a-day increase okayed by Dr. Podosin seemed to hold them at bay.

By June, I took Stephanie to see Dr. David Agnew, a neurologist located in Santa Barbara. We no longer had to travel to Los Angeles. He rekindled the hope in us that Stephanie could continue to learn and make progress. He explained some of her behavioral traits to me. A logical consequence led from impairment to conduct. I began to understand why Stephanie ignored her right side and constantly had to be reminded to use her right hand.

"When the body has suffered damage in a specific place, it doesn't want to entrust this faulty part to carry out anything it is charged to do. In Stephanie's case it is her right hand, her short-term memory loss, and her disorientation. The body starts to ignore this faulty circuit and bypasses it. You can see this when Stephanie ignores her right hand, or when she gets lost. But, there is hope! Stephanie can still be retrained. Plus there are new medicines on the market, and actually, there is a lot of hope. A great deal of research covering all areas of the brain is going on.

"I'd like to have Stephanie undergo a sleep-deprived EEG within the next few weeks, and depending on the outcome of that, I might send her to LA to a hospital to be monitored for seizures. What they do in the hospital is very exact. Stephanie would wear a sensored hat at all times that would detect even the smallest seizure. Seizures that would escape our observation now."

Stephanie imagined herself wearing this contraption. "A sensored hat?" She giggled. "Like a space cadet?"

The vision made all three of us break out laughing.

Later, Dr. Agnew measured the strength in Stephanie's hands. Her left measured 80 pounds, her right 25 pounds. Her pulse rate equaled that of an athlete: 60. Her blood pressure read 117 over 75. All normal. And this was the girl who had suffered a cardiac arrest!

Stephanie looked forward to the night of movies preceding the sleep-deprived EEG. I rented videos and watched them with her to keep her awake. The first few hours were fun, but after four in the morning, it was hard to stay awake—especially since she was not allowed to drink anything containing caffeine.

At the Santa Barbara Writers' Conference in late June, I met Dr. Perie Longo, poet and therapist. I told her Stephanie's story, and she said, Yes, she would be willing to help Stephanie with her problems, with her sadness, and with her writing of poetry.

The two met and connected immediately at an unknown, deeper level. Stephanie had disliked psychotherapy the few times she'd gone years ago, but these sessions were different. With Perie she played with words, put her dreams on paper, and gave expression to thoughts that pleased or pained her.

The loss of her relationship with her father still troubled Stephanie deeply. She never did express her anger fully to me. Only that one time—when she told me she wanted to swim to Anacapa—did she let me know of her profound sadness. The poetry sessions with Perie enabled her to make use of words expressing her anger, as in the poem, "Anger begins when nobody listens. "

Stephanie began to heal emotionally by writing poetry. She became more cheerful and seemed to adjust to her father being a remote figure from her past.

When Stephanie wrote poetry in my house, I usually transcribed her writing the moment she read the poem to me. Stephanie was gifted in expressing moods and meaning, and read with proper stops and commas, using the right intonations. But if I found one of her poems later, without the benefit of her reading, it would take time and effort to decipher her scrawly, unpunctuated script.

With Perie, Stephanie had begun to heal her wounded little girl's heart. And she wrote poem after poem. As she wrote, she simultaneously read it aloud, and Perie at that time would enter Steff's poem into her computer. Perie then handed Stephanie a printout of the poem. Sometimes Stephanie wanted Perie to substitute a different word that expressed her meaning more closely. When I picked her up from her lessons—her therapy—Stephanie always presented me with a gift I would come to value more than anything else, each Monday, her latest poem.

And so another *teacher* had come into Stephanie's life, as important to her at this stage as Marianne Frostig had been at an earlier one. Stephanie lost her sadness in these weeks, her seizures came under control, and she was writing, writing, writing.

Loneliness begins when I'm alone
In my bedroom.
I feel like a spot on the wall.
Sometimes I feel loneliness is
not having any friends
or a father who really cares.
Loneliness ends with tears
at night before
I go to bed.

Anger begins when nobody listens
to what I have to say.
I like throwing things to get my anger out.
Just once I'd like to throw my words out.
Earthquake!
Tidal Wave!
Volcano!
Red!
Purple, Black and Blue!
FATHER, listen to me NOW.
I mean RIGHT NOW.
Why don't you call me

Or write to me
Or see me more often.
It doesn't take that long to get to here
From L.A.

—Stephanie Finell, July 27, 1994

August came, and Stephanie spent a few days with Hugi, Brian, and their new baby, Jillian, in Los Angeles. When I picked her up, Hugi took me aside. "Karin," she whispered, "Stephanie had this really weird dream. Very disturbing. She dreamed she had died and was in heaven. Scared me half to death when she told me."

Suddenly I shivered. My body went cold. Very cold. I stared at Hugi, wondering if she had exaggerated. Just then Stephanie waltzed in from the bedroom, baby Jillian in her arms. "I don't want to go home," she said. "If I have to, I'd like to take Jillian along, she's such a love."

Later, in the car, I asked her if she remembered the dream that so upset Hugi. "Oh, Hugi. She gets upset over nothing. I told her I was in heaven, and it was beautiful. I was floating, and dancing, and I could use both my hands. Both my hands! I wasn't handicapped any more. To tell you the truth, I hated waking up, it was such a wonderful feeling being over there. But when I told Hugi, she got all weirded out. . .started crying. . .Really, Mom, it was only a dream."

I took Stephanie along to an appointment with my lawyer. I wanted Rob Laney to get to know Stephanie personally, because she was the principal beneficiary of my trust. But all this planning of what would happen after my death upset Stephanie. She grew pensive, her eyes misted. "Mom," she said, "What would I do without you? You can't leave me, Mom, you can't. I couldn't live—"

"Stephanie, these things are far off in the future. Don't worry, I'll be around for quite a while."

"Mom," her voice was a throaty whisper. "I'd like for both of us to go together, so no one would be left alone—"

"Don't talk nonsense, sweetie. It's nature's course that I will die before you. But I hope that by that time you'll have found someone you'll love, someone responsible."

"No one will ever look out for me the way you do."

I stroked her hair and handed her a tissue. She was giving voice to my own fears.

A few days later, Stephanie was at my house when she had a small seizure. I ran her a soothing warm bath, lit candles, played one of her favorite CDs of Native American flute music. She ducked under the water. Then her face emerged, wet and red, pearling water beads. "Mom," she said smiling, with that lilt of a question in her voice, "Can't you give me that picture there?" She pointed to a gouache of a blue nude facing us on the wall.

"Stephanie, I like that painting. . .it's perfect where it hangs. You don't have any wall-space for it in your house."

"I love it. I so want to look at it."

"You can look at it whenever you're here. I'll put a sticker on it, so after I die, it's yours."

"I don't want you to die, Mom, please. . .promise. . .I can't stand it." She shook and grabbed my arm as if in a small seizure and dug her nails into my skin. *Why did I make that thoughtless remark, when I knew that lately she had worried about life without me?*

"My little love," I said. "You can have the picture. But all in time. First I'll have to get something else for that wall." Stephanie shook her head. A tear, looking like a small glass bauble, slid down her wet face. "Stephanie, don't worry, both of us are going to live for a very long time."

"Sure?" She swallowed hard. Her eyes were wide now, reflecting the glow of the candles in her pupils. Stephanie. To me she was incredibly beautiful at that moment. My heart constricted with loving her so much.

Then she said, "I don't know Mom, sometimes I just don't know—"

"My melancholy princess. Cheer up. No more talk of dark subjects. The case is closed."

"Ha! Now you sound like Dad," she giggled. She grabbed me to plant a kiss, I almost lost my balance, seated as I was on the edge of the tub, but managed not to tumble into the water.

The idea of predeceasing a handicapped child is frightening for a parent. I discussed this with others in similar situations. Some of the disabled had siblings who would look after them when the parents died. Some did not. But even with responsible relatives, leaving a dependent child for others to care for is a terrible worry. Trust money does not compensate, and no one would love the child as unselfishly as a parent.

I held Stephanie in my eyes and hoped I'd live for a long, long time.

Chapter Twenty-Seven

Navajo Land

Sometimes I feel different like
An Indian maiden with feathers
hanging down. . . .
                    —Stephanie Finell

Late Summer, 1994

Stephanie heard me talk to Aida about longing to visit the American Southwest, my beloved landscape. She chimed right in and said, "Mom, why don't you take me with you. I'd love to see all that too and meet the Navajos; meet the friends you made."

"Steff, I go there to interview people and take notes. I'm working there; I'll be busy."

"I can be quiet. As quiet as a mouse. Please, Mom, please?

We flew to Albuquerque, rented a car, and drove to the Navajo Reservation near Gallup, New Mexico. I would renew my spirit among red rocks and rabbit brush, clear my lungs and mind, inhale the scent of cedar and pine, and take solace from the wide-open skies. Maybe the land would do the same for Stephanie? For just a little while I hoped to banish my fears of the future.

I hoped we could stay at the Franciscan Mission of St. Michaels, near the Navajo capital, Window Rock, or to be more precise, that we could stay at the adjacent convent, where I knew that the nuns, the teachers, were still on holiday.

Father Simon, the priest at the Mission whom I had become friends with when I was there earlier, greeted us with open arms.

He smiled, saying, "Of course you can stay at the convent."

Yes, I was right, the convent building was empty, and all we had to do was put the linens on our beds. I knew where the linen closets were, and we helped ourselves to bedclothes and towels. We would wash the linens before we left and leave the convent as we found it. Father Simon told the caretaker to see to it that the water heater was turned on for our showers. The sextant took us across the parking lot to the convent. The convent's kitchen carried a supply of instant coffee and tea, and some other nonperishables. We would eat breakfast there but join the Brothers and Father Simon for lunch and dinner, with an occasional break in the routine while visiting Tom and Marie Yazzie, my Navajo friends.

Father Simon was delighted finally to meet Stephanie, of whom I had spoken so many times on previous visits.

The first evening, as we walked the empty hallways of the convent, Stephanie pressed close to my side and said, "Isn't it spooky, Mom?"

I shook my head. "Not to me it isn't. Come on, let's make our beds."

The rooms were small, each holding one narrow bed, a small desk and a chair plus a narrow wardrobe. "Mom, I don't want to sleep by myself. Can't we move another bed in here and sleep in the same room?"

"There really isn't room for it—"

I was interrupted by a knock at the door." Yes, come in—"

It was the caretaker carrying our luggage.

"Ask him," Steffi nudged me. "Ask him if there's a larger room?"

The sextant answered Stephanie in a soft voice, "Oh yes, there is a larger room used by the Mother Superior. We haven't had one now for a few years. I'm sure it would be alright if you moved into that room."

He left with our suitcases, and off he went, down the long hallway and down the stairs, and we followed, to arrive at a bright room with two beds, a dressing table or desk, and two upholstered chintz chairs. A perfect room for the two of us.

But after a good night's sleep, we awakened with growling stomachs. I knew we'd have to go to the market to buy milk and eggs and bread if we were to breakfast in the convent. It made more sense on this day to accept the invitation for breakfast at the Mission. There a hearty meal was laid out. Several of the Brothers had taken their seats. The cook had cereals and eggs and bacon and toast lined up on a rolling cart. Coffee steamed from two carafes. Butter, honey, and jams sat on the long table, and each person helped himself. Stephanie was hungry, and she dug right in without waiting for anyone to bless the food first. It was my fault, I had not told her to wait until she observed what everyone was going to do. When I lived with my grandmother I was accustomed to saying grace before a meal, but all those gracious manners were forgotten in the harried pace of Los Angeles. I now felt it was a lovely way of saying, *thank you* for all that was provided for us, and here at the Mission, where it came from the heart, it touched me. I couldn't explain Stephanie's behavior to the Brothers, who had probably thought we were devout Catholics. Stephanie put her fork down the moment she caught my eye and noticed she had committed a faux pas.

Stephanie made friends easily, even here with the Franciscan Brothers. Eighty-five-year-old Brother Francis became her favorite. He took us on a long trek to an ancient Anasazi house built high up on a cliff. I am afraid of heights, and Stephanie would not be able to climb, and only he was brave enough to scale up. I worried that if anything happened to him, neither one of us would be able to help him. But he went up the cliff like a mountain goat and pointed out the decaying mud houses blending in with the surrounding cliff, which were built in the thirteenth century by the people who were the ancestors of the present-day Pueblo and Hopi Indians.

Then there was Brother John, whom Steffi called *Frère Jacques,* even singing the nursery rhyme of his name in French. He organized the weekly bingo game and when Thursday arrived, both Stephanie and I helped him with the cards and the ticket sales.

The following day, Father Simon suggested he would take us to the flea market in Gallup. We were overwhelmed with the variety of local handcrafted goods. Many of the pottery items were made in the Pueblos around Santa Fe; others in the village of Zuni, near Gallup. Stephanie kept fingering a lovely Zuni fetish necklace, made with turquoise-and-white shell and cornelian. I bought it for her. She should have a nice memory of her first visit to this land of magic.

In the evening when I was already in bed, she came over to me, holding the necklace, saying, "Mom, this would really look nice on you."

"But I bought it for you, Stephanie."

"I know. But I want you to have it. Nobody buys you things any more. May I borrow it some time?"

Stephanie's tenderness never failed to touch me. Sometimes I wondered if she would be this caring, this sensitive, if she were not in some ways disabled? If she had not been struck by encephalitis, would she have been more self-centered—as I was at her age? Was her incredible sweetness-of-being a compensation for the deep sadness that she was not *whole*? In some ways, I reminded myself, she was *more than whole*.

Some people envied me. They told me how lucky I was to have Stephanie accompany me to faraway places. I would squint my eyes and bite my lip. Did these people have any idea how difficult it was to face someone you loved so much, day after day, to realize over and over again that she would never reach the potential she was born with? Your child, who would always need to be protected? How could I make them understand I would be happier if she were able to attend a university. If she were married to someone with whom she could have a child. I would be happier if Stephanie were independent.

Still I had to admit, there was some truth in their remarks. Traveling with Stephanie was a small compensation. I was grateful that so far I still had the funds to afford it. During our travels, I forgot worries about our future—worries about when my money would run out—worries of repeated seizure attacks. (Stephanie had never had a seizure on a major trip with me, only that one time in Chattanooga where we were with the entire family followed by the days in Florida.) Travel served to teach her much about the world and its varied people, things she could not learn by reading books. We were happy on our trips. But during those times when Stephanie showed awareness of her condition, the deep ache within me would always surface again.

A few days after our excursion to Gallup, Father Simon said, "If Stephanie were Navajo and had suffered this disease, her awareness wouldn't have been affected nearly as much. Living with extended families in a more basic society would have enabled her to fit in."

I thought of Stephanie's time spent with my friends in Guadalajara, Mexico, and how she adjusted to life there—and seemingly belonged. I regretted that our "advanced" society was so excluding.

One day when we visited Tom and Marie Yazzie, a Navajo family who had befriended me on my previous visits, Tom surprised us with his plan to take us and his two granddaughters to Canyon de Chelly, to visit his *Bima Sani*, his grandmother, nearby and then go to Monument Valley.

We piled into his truck, and he drove to places where legends abound. On the way we met a woman who was almost a hundred years old and still actively weaving small carpets on her loom. In fact she cut one off the loom and gave it to me as a present. Stephanie was speechless. We drove to see Spider Woman's Rock in Canyon de Chelly, and Tom told us the legend of the ever industrious female spider who was the preserver of the hearth and taught weaving to the women of *Dinétah*—Navajo women. This legend tied right in with the grandmother whom we had just visited. She would be industrious until her life ended.

The day passed quickly, and we still had many miles to drive to Monument Valley. This time I would not feel like a tourist, now we were part of a Navajo family and this after all was *Dinétah*—Navajo country. Stephanie had seen my photographs, and I had read her pages from my book in progress, but the reality of the place and its wondrous formations of red rock do not find space to breathe on a paper page. The shifting light in this wide open space cannot be described. How it illuminated the strange rock formations and its shadows transformed them into myths.

It was growing late, and typical for this time of year, storm clouds neared. The sky spoke, and the first drop of rain interrupted my thoughts. Nature rewarded us with a wild thundershower. First, huge dark clouds sailed the blue-green sky, changing to violet and to a charcoal gray above us. It was early evening, and the low sun and its orange red behind the clouds turned the horizon to magenta and purple. Lightning flashed and thunder spoke directly above us, and a downpour enveloped us in a warm shower. Stephanie, as I anticipated, loved it. Tom was much impressed that she did not, as most tourists would, run for shelter in the visitors' center.

The days flew by. We had our last meal of Navajo fry bread with Tom and Marie Yazzie and their family. Our suitcases were packed, and we were ready to leave. Father Simon took us into the chapel he had designed in the shape of a hogan, a traditional Navajo home built in the round with the door facing toward the rising sun. Here he prayed for our safe return home. We went to the dining room and thanked the cook who was clearing the table. We cast one last look at the kitchen, where we had helped the Brothers with the dishes—like ever so many fast automatons, but alive and giggling in their routine, and often singing while they worked.

The time had come to say goodbye to these friendly Brothers, and to give another big hug to Father Simon, this man who was so natural and loving to every human being. He played songs from the 1960s on his guitar for Stephanie and often sang Hank Williams ballads. Now he took us to our rental car, and we waved goodbye through the window. The large red brick church, St. Michaels Mission, reminiscent of British churches from the late nineteenth century, grew smaller in the rearview mirror, and sadness crept back into my eyes.

And then we bid a loving farewell to the open landscape. Stephanie looked wistful when she said, "I will miss it, Mom. Thanks for taking me along. I was good, wasn't I?"

"Yes, you were—" I said as I blew my runny nose.

"And the skies at night, the many stars, and it's so clear. Doesn't it remind you a little bit of Africa?"

"Yes, Stephanie, it does. It's the high desert, the clear air, the wide skies. You are so right." I wanted to lean over and kiss her, but the road was a two-lane highway, and one always had to look out for a stray dog—or maybe a horse bolting across the road.

Here I had the feeling of being at one with the universe—of being an unimportant speck in this nature that allowed a glimpse into forever. It was all here, in Navajo land, much as it had been in East Africa. Stephanie had begun to share my love for the Southwest. I hoped this would be the first of many trips with her to this place of enchantment.

I AM A WHOLE PERSON
I am not a roof on top of the house
I am a feather, a bright blue feather

I am not a hip acting chick
I am a note on a guitar
I am a whole person
a deep person
I am not cheap ordinary small things
you find at the mall like girls
who think small, not bright
who think only boys and money and sex

Sometimes I feel different like
An Indian maiden with feathers
hanging down.
I hate to think Indians had to die
from white people like me, at that time.
Sometimes I feel guilty
though I didn't kill them
I feel privileged to know them
to have them know I am
not a bad person
that I respect their ways
When they teach me to act
a certain way
while in their home.

I am not a tower on fire
I am not a mountain being blown by the wind

We must respect the earth.

—Stephanie Finell, September 19, 1994

Chapter Twenty-Eight

Falling in Love Again

You are sweet, genuine.
I felt I could fly.
    —Stephanie Finell

Fall 1994

It was one of those golden days in October, when air and water still carry within the warmth of summer.

Martin, Stephanie, and I, and Capri also were swimming at East Beach. The sun hung low. We were floating on our backs in smooth seas, and the water reflected the light with a bronze sheen.

Stephanie kept throwing the stick for Capri, delighted when Capri swam way beyond the second tier of waves, surfing with stick in muzzle. But after several throws Capri didn't return to Steff in the water, but approached a suntanned and muscular blond man crouching in the sand. He grabbed the stick and threw it far out for her to fetch again. He obviously liked dogs. Or perhaps the dog's owner?

"Mom, I'm cold," Stephanie said as she ran out, shaking off shimmering drops and wrapping herself in a Snoopy towel. I watched as the young man edged over and talked to her. They stood close now, with Stephanie tilting her face, hair dripping, feet shoveling sand. Her stance seemed shy and awkward. He asked a question. Capri stood wagging her tail, then tried to dig a hole to hide her stick, spraying an arc of sand. The young man pulled a flask from his backpack. I watched as Steff cupped her hands, and I saw him pour liquid into her upturned palms. Capri, snout up, pink tongue hanging, eyed this maneuver, but then, Steff hopped back and the fluid ran like quicksilver through her fingers. Both now stood looking silly, holding their sides with laughter. He then handed the thermos to Stephanie. She poured—what I guessed to be water—into his cupped hands, and Capri lapped it up.

Later, when I joined them, he explained, "That was ice water—that's why your daughter jumped."

He was polite, seemed nice. And he liked dogs. "My name is Duane," he said, and asked, "And yours?"

"I'm Stephanie." He asked for her phone number. Steff was quick to tell him that she was in the phone book, the only S. Finell listed.

On Sunday, their first date, he picked her up from my house where Stephanie spent her weekends when Aida visited friends in Los Angeles. Stephanie bubbled over when she came home.

"He's so polite, opened the door for me. He took me to such a nice restaurant, Mom, and to a movie. He's wonderful, just wonderful. Don't you think he has the nicest eyes? Blue, no green. And I love his sun-streaked hair."

He did have nice eyes, though I detected a sadness in them. He worked as a carpenter, nearby, and had not lived in Santa Barbara for long. And typically, I worried again. I knew I mustn't be such a proverbial mother hen. Stephanie was a young woman, and she had been married. But then, she was not like other young women her age; she was a child-woman. She needed protection. Something in her would never grow up, perhaps that was part of her charm. Duane on the other hand was nine years older and had been divorced for several years.

All this didn't matter to Stephanie. Her unending subject of conversation from this moment on was *Duane*, wonderful Duane.

In the beginning Stephanie worried that Duane might lose interest in her. "I'm such a dork. He won't like me for long," she said.

I tried to give her confidence. How could she call herself a dork?

The next time he picked her up, they went to Hendry's Beach. They built a sand castle. She told me it was huge, and they decorated it with driftwood and shells and bits of rope and used a piece of tee shirt as a flag. All day they stayed at the beach, swimming, walking, and playing in the sand. She told me this was one of the best days in her life. Later she wrote this poem:

WE PADDLED TO SHORE
We gathered seashells
We built a sandcastle
A very high sandcastle
Taller than a child
Beautiful.
So many shapes and colors
Like out of a fairytale.
Like a dream.

Some of the sand was wet,
some dry. Some mixed.

On top we put a heart-shaped rock,
which meant I liked you.
You are sweet, genuine.
I felt I could fly.
Up to a shining star.
I felt I would cry.

We walked to the other side of the point.
I made my wish.
I don't know if you'll stay. . .
I'm scared to talk about it.
I'm not sure you'll call again.
I think you've had a lot of sadness.
A lot of sadness.
When you said goodbye
You did not look into my eyes.

—Stephanie Finell, October 9, 1994

And then, seemingly having detected a similar sadness in Duane's eyes as I had earlier, she wrote this poem:

SOMETHING'S MISSING
I need a long term relationship
I see a sadness
in his eyes
like he's missing his old life.
I think he needs love
and tenderness.
Inside me something's missing too.
There is an emptiness
though we talk.
He has his work. He has me.

He loves to spend time on the beach
with me. Could it be
after the New Year
he might live with me.
I would love it.
I would love it.

—Stephanie Finell, October 24, 1994

When earlier she had said, *I'm not sure he'll call again*, her assumption turned out to be wrong. He did call again. And again. They saw each other almost every day. He drove a van, and those days when he picked her up from my house, he always brought her back at the precise hour he promised. He talked about a sailboat, partially built, which he hoped to finish soon. This boat—a forty-three-foot Ferro-concrete sloop—was still in Sacramento, where Duane used to live.

"Concrete? Won't that boat sink? " I asked.

"No way." He shook his head emphatically. "Boats are made of iron, of cement, of all kinds of material. It's the design that keeps her afloat. Steff and I will sail around the Caribbean. Right, Steff? She loves the water, ole Scorpio girl."

"You're a Scorpio too," Stephanie said.

"Yep. And we both love the water." He put his arm around her, giving her a squeeze. "We'll just sail, and sail, right into the sunset."

"That's very nice, but what are you going to buy the groceries with?"

"I'm working. I'll save up some money. It'll work out. Right, Steff?"

"Right. It'll be such fun, Mom. I miss our boat. You know I love sailing."

I kept my tongue in check. After all, his boat was far from being finished. I didn't have to worry. Not yet.

Duane treated Stephanie with tenderness. And she blossomed, like a sunflower opening its petals to the light. She smiled and sang and danced. One day I noticed her writing, then she abruptly put the yellow pad and pencil aside and moved the fingers of her right hand as if she were remembering the hand gestures from her former dancing instructions. A little later I found her poem:

> I can move my bad hand like a rose,
> like a butterfly,
> like a snake.
> I can dance with my hand.

During that time, in the early weeks of October 1994, Stephanie underwent a battery of tests administered by a psychologist. I was given an oral explanation and also a written evaluation of her capabilities. The written one stated what goals might be attainable and which were out of reach.

We saw Dr. Agnew again. When he read in the report that Stephanie would *never* drive a car, he shook his head, smiled and said, "Never say *never*. We're dealing with the brain, and much is uncharted territory. What we know about the brain currently is what has been discovered within the last five or ten years. There is a lot of hope, still."

He was a caring man, and I felt lucky to have found a doctor who gave us hope. Dr. Agnew scheduled a PET scan for Steff in Los Angeles at USC

General Hospital, on Friday, November 4, since there was no Positron Emission Tomography machine in Santa Barbara yet. The multicolored images of the brain gave doctors a reading of the biological health of the organ at the cellular level. It would be quite a procedure, but afterward we would know the geography of Stephanie's brain, where it was scarred and which part was functioning. The PET scan images would be a map, a guide to show the location of the areas where progress could take place. It would also chart where Stephanie's seizures were located. These were peculiar now; she seemed to be talking in tongues, *Kam-chatka, kam-chatka, kam-chatka*—

I spoke to Duane of her illness, and of her present problem. He had to know, in case Stephanie acted, as she would say, "weird." He took the information in stride, as if seizures were a normal part of life.

The date for the PET scan arrived, and we drove to downtown Los Angeles, to one of the USC hospital sites. Stephanie had asked Duane to come along. On our way, we stopped at Hamburger Hamlet, a restaurant near Marvin's condo, where Stephanie introduced Duane to her father. It would be lunchtime soon, and we were all hungry, but we had to help Stephanie with her will power—she was not allowed to eat for six hours prior to the test. And so we too subdued our appetite and only drank coffee. It made Stephanie happy to read approval of Duane in her father's eyes. She quenched her thirst with water and, for the moment, forgot all about food.

I said goodbye to her as she lay on a steel table with dyed fluids running through her veins, while a color-screen monitor scanned her brain. In the waiting room, Duane stretched his arm to check his watch, paced the room, and finally suggested that he and I take the elevator down to the cafeteria and grab a bite to eat. It took longer than anticipated. I knew Stephanie would be hungry and ordered a slice of pizza and a drink to take up to her.

When we finally arrived on Stephanie's floor, we found her sitting in the waiting room, with tears streaming down her face. She got up and shouted in Duane's face, "You! You didn't keep your promise, Duane! You didn't wait! You too, Mom!"

They had finished the test earlier than expected. The nurse and the receptionist had left for the weekend, only the technician who administered the scan was still in the office.

Stephanie was right. We should have waited for her in the reception room.

"Steffi, don't be such a ninny. We were back when we thought you'd be finished. How could we know you'd be done that soon?" Duane said.

"You promised you wouldn't go anywhere. You'd wait for me. Right here. What could I do if you didn't come back?"

"Silly, we wouldn't just leave you here," I said.

"They were locking up the place." She wiped her eyes.

"Come on. Snap out of it. Here, have some pizza," Duane said.

She pushed his hand with the pizza away, but she reached for the Coke.

Duane put his arm around her and led her out the door. He didn't know Stephanie well enough to understand her fear. He couldn't imagine the overwhelming helplessness she must have felt, knowing she would never be able to find us in this large hospital, knowing she had no way of getting home alone. Duane could not conceive the extent of her dependency. I knew I was to blame, for not having given her a booklet with telephone numbers of her father and our friends in Los Angeles. How much easier life is now with cell phones.

Yet, in some ways, Duane treated her and any particular situation in just the right way. He always remained calm and unruffled, as if Stephanie's seizures were part of her and were to be treated as nature's little temblor. The kind when she gazes into space and talks in tongues, as she had done in Ojai. When it happened at a Von's market, the girl at the checkout stand had stared. Duane, in a cool voice said, "She's having a seizure. Do you have a problem with that?" When Stephanie told me about it later, I thought he handled it very well. And I was glad he'd been forewarned.

PET SCAN
I was scared to go in
actually.
I ate at 7:00.
Duane came at 9:00, right on time.
It took my Mom one hour
and fifteen minutes to get to LA.
Before the PET scan
we visited our old home.
The big one on Ridgedale Drive.
All these strange people mobbed
around our car. I had to visit
my father. That's where the weird looking
people, strange people, were.
Luckily we had a man to protect us.
Duane. The PET scan took two-and-a-half
hours. A couple of times I got scared.
A black guy in white came in,
took some x-rays, told me to stretch out.
I don't want to experience it again.
The thumping reminds me of getting
my teeth done.
I was so hungry.
I was dreaming of pizza.
When I came out no one was there.
Mom and Duane had gone out to eat.
I was alone, frightened. But,

I'd wait for Duane forever.
I'm happy I saw my father alone.
Without her. He wants me to be happy
With someone I can love.
He said, "Keep up the good work."

—Stephanie Finell, November 1994

(Introducing Duane to her father made her nervous. There were no people who "mobbed" the car. The PET scan took less than one and a half hours. She saw her father alone because Judith had the flu.)

I overheard Stephanie tell Duane how good it felt when she sat behind the wheel of a car. "Some people like flying an airplane, well, to me driving was like that. I felt so free. The landscape swooshing past me—"

"You must' a gone too fast then."

"No. I kept to the speed limit. But driving. . .it's such a wonderful feeling. If only I knew someone who would teach me how to drive again. It's been a while. I'd have to pass the test for a new learner's permit again."

After that request, Duane began teaching her the driving rules from the DMV book. It was as if the two were playing school. He told her a rule, she repeated it; then he questioned her about those rules, making her repeat the ones she had a hard time remembering, as in, *What is a soft shoulder?*

The third time she giggled and answered: "Mom's." I could see her eyes twinkle behind the spread of her fingers. Continuing in earnest, she answered correctly, "When the side next to the road you're on is not paved? Like with gravel or something?"

"Right."

And on went the lessons.

I made it clear to Duane that Stephanie wouldn't be able to drive until her seizures were under control. He nodded and went right on drilling her with rules and regulations.

Stephanie was wild about Duane, and it worried me that he had such power over her. When he hinted he might come over for lunch, nothing could make her stir from the house. There she would be, waiting for him, wearing a smile. He often brought a ready-to-eat meal, or he cooked for both of them. Her solicitous behavior concerned me, but I let it go, for I had never seen her so radiant before. She told me she had never known love like this before. This all-consuming feeling of being on top of the world. Love.

I asked her if she had forgotten Loren? Or how she felt when she first met Loren? She smiled her enigmatic Mona Lisa smile. "I thought I was in love with Loren, but, Mom, I didn't really know love then. And Loren, I still love the guy, but differently, more like a brother."

Now she was a *woman* in love and felt Duane loved her back. But it was more than that. It was as if a dam had opened, and the flood of water rushing out was inundating all reason. I was afraid she might get into a situation where she would lose control.

She did whatever Duane wanted her to do. He was polite to me, and whenever Steff became sassy, which happened once in a while, he told her to apologize and show respect to her mother. I had no obvious reason to be troubled, but this young man remained an enigma to me. He never talked about himself, his past, or his family. After seeing a lot of him for almost two months, I knew no more about him than on the first day we met him. But I knew my daughter, and any interference from me would cause her to rebel. I also was careful not to curb her happiness. I remembered the lines from William Blake: *He who binds to himself a joy / Doth the winged life destroy.*

We celebrated Stephanie's birthday on a Saturday with a "Scorpio party." Steffi and Duane, and several of the guests were all Scorpios. I rummaged through closets and returned with an armful of hats, some of them silly indeed. Some of fur, some with feathers, some from faraway places, such as Ladakh, India. Each of us put on a hat and voilà! We felt in a party mood. Duane, who wore his hat backward made Stephanie shriek with laughter when its long pheasant feather dipped into his salad. The candles were lit on a cake with the Scorpio guests' names written in purple icing, and the cake was decorated with crawly chocolate scorpions.

On Stephanie's actual birthday, Duane took her to dine at romantic Cold Spring Tavern, an old stagecoach stop up the mountain pass. When he picked her up from my house, he arrived with a long golden box, and when Stephanie opened it, she found two dozen long-stemmed roses in it. Red roses. A sentimental card accompanied the flowers. Stephanie buried her face in the soft petals, saying, "They're beautiful, Duane, but—"

"But what?"

"Soon they will be dead."

A few weeks later, we drove Aida to the airport. She wept sad tears for leaving Stephanie behind, and happy tears in anticipation of seeing her family in Guatemala. Later that evening, Steff took me aside. "Mom. . .?"

"Yes?"

"I've been thinking about this for a long time. I hope you understand. When Aida comes back in January, I would like for her to live with you. I want to live by myself and be more independent."

"But you need her to help you out with—"

"That's just the problem. She's always there to help me out. I never get to do things, or even try to do them on my own. Give me a chance, Mom."

"Does Duane have anything to do with this idea?"

"Well?" Her lips spread in a lopsided half-smile, as if gauging my response. "Yes. I'm so happy with him, when we're alone. You know, on the weekends, when Aida goes to LA. By the way, I made an omelet the other day all by myself." She giggled. "But you know what I did? I put it on the griddle instead of in a pan. It was delicious anyway. Duane liked it, but he said. . .never mind."

"What did he say?"

"I could have started a major fire. But that's not true, just some of the egg-stuff ran down the burners."

"It's lucky you have an electric stove. I don't know what would have happened in my house with gas. Stephanie, it's too dangerous for you to live alone. I have to think about this. I mean. . .the idea scares me. If. . .now I haven't agreed to anything yet, but, if I okayed this arrangement, I'd want you to keep Capri with you. And I would want you to call me every morning before you go to your school. *And* when you come back."

"Mom, you worry too much. Let me be free."

"I worry because you still get lost. And I don't want Duane to live with you when you're not married. That you have to promise. He can visit you there, but I'd like for him to keep his own apartment."

"Then you would let Aida stay with you? Would you? Yes? That would be so cool. I love Aida, but I can't learn anything with her around."

I smiled sadly, knowing her statement was true.

In the following weeks, with Aida gone, I found Duane kind and firm with Stephanie. He made her do her own laundry, fold clothes properly; he made her vacuum, and tidy up. In fact, after two weeks the house looked as clean as if Aida were still there. Stephanie was very proud of the fact that she was finally learning to keep house.

Stephanie and Duane spent Christmas Eve by themselves. She told me they sat by candlelight in front of the fireplace, with lights twinkling on the little tree they had bought together and decorated.

Early Christmas morning, I heard Duane's van come up our driveway. Stephanie, dressed in Christmas red, jumped out. Capri followed. Stephanie hugged me, hugged Martin, and then rushed into the house, eager to unwrap presents.

She ripped open the silver wrapping of her brother's present first. A musical snow-crystal ball enclosing an angel appeared from the paper, and the box played "Für Elise," by Beethoven. Stephanie wept with joy. (How curious, it was the same piece of music she had played on the piano when she first came back from the hospital, almost twenty-three years before.) From that moment onward she carried the snow-crystal angel with her wherever she went.

Cousin Tracy and our friend Allan joined us for dinner. Logs crackled in the hearth, garlands of pine festooned with red bows circled the windows and wound around the dining room's chandelier. Yes, ours was a cozy Christmas.

Later, before sleep came, I reflected upon Stephanie's life. She had overcome so many obstacles. I was content, for she now had reached a high point in her life. She wrote poetry with increasing fervor and intensity. She was conscientious with her volunteer job—working with children fulfilled her. It made her feel wanted and needed. She lived in her own little cottage with a beautiful garden and was learning how to take care of her home. In Duane she had found a man she loved, a man who made her feel complete. Other than still missing her father, there was nothing in the world that could add to the happiness that filled her that Christmas. And grateful for her life, I fell asleep.

Chapter Twenty-Nine

Spirit Visit

I swim amid the Seas of Loving Kindness
As nature goes its many ways. . .
      —Stephanie Finell, January 7, 1995

Ojai, January 7, 1995

Saturday arrived too quickly. This was our last day at the Oaks' mother and daughter week.

The day dawned gray when Stephanie crept into my bed, snuggling close. She nudged me, "Mom, Grandma was here again this morning."

"Grandma? You dreamed of her again?"

"No, not a dream. I saw her. She came and sat at the foot of my bed—"

My mother? Why didn't she appear to me, when there was so much we hadn't resolved? I shook my head. "What did she look like? What did she say?"

"She looked beautiful, sort of shiny, all in white. She said she loved me and she would be there for me."

"Maybe she's your guardian angel now. She'll protect you from seizures."

"I won't have any more seizures. Not now. . .not with Duane loving me."

"Stephanie, you had one a while ago, with him right there by your side at Von's market. Remember?"

"That was then. This is now. I'm more in love with him every day, and soon I'll be strong and seizure free. 'Love cures all,' Duane said." Her eyes had taken on a dreamy, gazing-into-the-future look as she leaned over and gave me a big kiss.

Then she scooted down lower below the sheets, put her head on my shoulder and with her left hand pulled the blanket up. "Tell me, Mom, were you in love, very much in love when you met Dad?"

"You know I was. I told you that."

"Tell me again. How did you two meet?"

"Actually I met him through your grandmother."

"Grandma? She introduced you?"

"No, but I went with her to her lawyer, about a lawsuit she had. Your dad came back from lunch, saw us sitting in the reception area, and asked the secretary to bring him our file. Ours was a silly. . .a piddly case. . .normally your father wouldn't have handled it." I smiled, remembering. "But he saw me. . .and then, it was love at first sight. Both for him—well, I thought so—but certainly for me. He asked Grandma formally, 'May I take your daughter out to dinner this weekend?' Imagine, he didn't ask me, but your grandma! So old-fashioned. He was brought up a southern gentleman. That was part of his charm."

"And. . .go on!"

Grandma said, "Why don't you ask my daughter?"

"Of course he did, and we had our first date at the Luau. The place was made for lovers. Hawaiian décor, perfumed candles on the tables, soft music. Then your dad asked me what I planned to do with my life. I told him I hoped to be a writer, and that I took evening classes at city college, English, and creative writing, and. . .well, he really paid attention. He listened." I smiled, remembering. "When he looked at me with his intense eyes, I couldn't eat a bite. And I'd been ravenous! God, I was so happy that this handsome, intelligent man cared about what I thought, and what I planned to do with my life. I got all misty eyed, emotional." Remembering, I had to grab a tissue again.

"Tell me more." Stephanie snuggled even closer.

"After dinner, your father took me dancing at L'Escoffier, the penthouse restaurant at the Beverly Hilton. He danced light on his feet and led me into swirls and turns I had not danced before." Stephanie looked wide-eyed and said, "Yes, I too love dancing with Dad. Go on, more, tell me more."

"Well, in the middle of a number, he stooped to pick up a half-opened rose lying on the dance floor, saying that this little flower should not be stepped on. That did it. The rose became a symbol. I was the rosebud, and he would be my protector, and no one would ever trample on me again. And that's how it all started."

"That's so romantic. . .And then what happened?" She looked at me with a growing sadness in her eyes. "I know—" She nodded as if in conversation with herself. Then she continued with questions that at the same time sounded like answers. "But. . .why did Dad drink so much? Was it me? Because I got my illness?"

"No, Stephanie." I stroked her hair, trying not to show my unhappiness. "Your father always drank a lot. When he was working in the law firm, and when he was younger, he could handle it. One circumstance led to the next. Don't feel responsible, please. Don't ever. . .But things did change after your illness. My own perceptions as to what is important and what is not, they certainly changed. So did your father's. We each experience pain and trauma at a different level,. . .and your father. . .I can't second-guess why he acted the way he did, why he drank in excess or did any of the things he did. All I know is why I changed."

Something in my relationship to Stephanie was revealed to me at that moment. Something I hadn't understood before. It astonished me to hear myself say, "Stephanie, I believe you became my teacher."

"Me? Your teacher?" She giggled. "Be serious!"

"Yes. You taught me how to really see. To go beyond the obvious. To delve deep, really deep, to the core of what *is*. You made me understand what is important in life, and what is not. How to be grateful for all the little things others take for granted." I paused, letting my hand glide over the softness of her cheek. "When you cross a street and see someone in a wheelchair, you always say, 'Thank you, God. Thank you, my Guardian Angel, that I have legs and am able to walk.' Stephanie, you always dwell on the positive, never on the 'poor me' aspect. And you taught me how to be aware of life around me. I live more intensely, and more in the present moment, all because of you."

"And I've done that?" Her eyes widened.

"Yes, you have, my little lovebug. But, hop-hop now. Out of bed! Breakfast is waiting, classes are waiting. We have to get dressed."

A minute or so later, while I slipped into my jogging pants, Stephanie appeared from the bathroom, toothbrush in hand, her mouth full of toothpaste. She hugged me hard. "Mom, I love you so much. So much. You are happy now, aren't you?"

"Yes, I am. What's more, I feel peaceful. Yes, with you and with Martin. . .and with our house and garden—"

"I'm sorry for Dad. That he can't see things as they are."

"He sees the same things we see, but he perceives a different reality."

"Sort of like someone who's colorblind? He sees red when it's green?"

I smiled, amazed at her insight. "Yes, something like that. But who's to say? Maybe his thoughts are right, and mine are wrong? Maybe it's really red, when I see green? How about that? Now rinse your mouth, Stephanie. You look like you have rabies."

The minute I uttered those words, the vision of the onset of her illness flashed into my mind—the foaming mouth. Rabies, another disease affecting the brain.

She trudged off and returned with a rinsed mouth and a piece of paper, saying, "Mom, I wrote to Dad last night. Want to read it? And a poem—"

I nodded. I took the paper from her hand and read: "Dear Father and Judy, I am going home Saturday. I can't wait to see my boyfriend Duane. I miss him so much—"

On the same sheet of her unfinished letter, some poetic thoughts followed:

I SWIM AMID THE SEAS OF LOVING KINDNESS
As nature goes its many ways
I've come to this conclusion
That God is perfect in all ways

He is the Ultimate
Who can do all
And know all
And we can see his work in nature

We tend to be obstinate
And not realize all things are ONE
All things are beautiful
All animals are beautiful
Lizards and snakes
All birds are beautiful
All chameleons,
All buffaloes are beautiful
Deer and mice are cute
Even though, most animals don't get along. . .

—Stephanie Finell, January 7, 1995

Even though, most animals don't get along. How true, Stephanie! This certainly applied to the human animal, when we look and see all the warring nations, and then shift our view down to the microcosm of many families. But there is hope, deer and mice are cute! Do they then get along? I smiled to myself, thinking of Stephanie's poem while we followed Maura the yoga teacher's instructions.

When it was time to relax, and everyone stretched out, Stephanie's hand inched over the carpet to touch mine. She squeezed my fingers. I glanced at her out of the corner of my eye and she mouthed, "I love you, Mom."

We returned to Santa Barbara that evening. Duane came to pick up Stephanie. They went back to her little house. We hugged longer than usual when we said goodbye.

On Monday I saw Stephanie briefly when I picked her up from Perie's poetry therapy. She had written this poem:

IF I HAD TO LIVE MY LIFE OVER
I would choose the same way
to show people how to deal with problems,
to not look down on yourself.

I feel I can accomplish more goals
in life with my illness
I don't need to learn to drive.
I feel more secure with Duane,
He's teaching me new things
like turning on the washing machine.
I can fold clothes, put them away
nice and neat. I used to say,
"Let Aida do it. . .Let Mom do it."
But now, *I do it.*
I'm positive in every respect.
He did it.
When I told him about my illness
he didn't leave.
He told me to talk in a good sense
about myself, not a bad sense.
He makes me see what I can do
with my life. He doesn't even look
at other women. That makes me feel
so special.
We go to movies.
He puts his arm around me
at night on the sofa in the rain.
It's so cozy, so romantic.
I'm so in love with him.
He says he loves me back

—Stephanie Finell, January 9, 1995

Chapter Thirty

Rainbows and Moonbows

"When you die, you will be spoken of as those in the sky, like the stars."

—Yurok proverb

Or, like the most wondrous of all, the moonbow

The end came without warning. Without signs. She stepped into the steaming tub, soaked, and sang as was her habit, then suddenly her voice was still. No sound, but for the water, drip by drip pulling through the drain.

The stillness alerted him. He opened the door to see if she was all right. The water had run out. She lay with her head touching her shoulder, lashes fanning her cheeks, and wet hair streaming over her face, a half smile on her lips.

He tried to revive her. Mouth to mouth, one more kiss. But she did not awaken as in a fairytale.

The paramedics arrived, and then the police.

And all that time I was alive. Perhaps I was watching television or reading a book. I knew Duane was with Stephanie, a man who loved her and with whom she would be safe during the torrential rains, these January floods with mud slides that blocked the road between our two houses.

How could I have slept? How could I not have known?

The call came at 9:30 a.m. A sheriff asked if he could come to see me. I thought he wanted to solicit funds and asked him to state his business over the phone.

"Are you alone?" he asked.

A strange question. "No, someone is with me," I said.

"Mrs. Finell, this concerns your daughter, Stephanie—"

My heart skipped a beat, a wave of cold washed over me. *Stephanie. Maybe she was hit by a car on her way to Peabody School?* I asked, "Was there an accident?"

"No, Mrs. Finell, your daughter—she's dead."

"Is what?"

"Your daughter died last night."

"*Whaaat?*" I might have heard the words but did not understand.

He repeated, "Your daughter died last night."

Silence. Then my shriek.

As from far, far away I heard him say, "That's why I wanted to come over Ma'am, to tell you in person. . .are you sure there's someone with you?"

Martin had taken the phone. I dimly heard him speaking to someone, *who?* while I sank onto the carpet.

Thoughts began to stir. Last night? Why had no one called me earlier?

I screamed and wept and could not comprehend. Stephanie dead? My vibrant, laughing Stephanie. No, this was a mistake.

Everything surrounding me seemed disconnected from reality. I looked out the window. The clouds were still holding up the sky, the wind still rustled the palms, the rabbit sat near its hiding bush munching grass. All things went on as they had before. But everything continued living in another plane of existence.

And you—lay dead

What happened?

A massive seizure killed Stephanie. Duane called 911. When the police came, summoned by the ambulance crew, they arrested him. In the early morning, they let him go, after the coroner determined that no foul play was involved.

I knew I had to pull myself out of my haze. I knew I had to function. And I did, like an automaton. Arrangements had to be made. Calls to Marvin, to Steven in St. Louis, to Aida, still in Guatemala. Martin called our friends. I asked Father Simon, from St. Michaels on the Navajo reservation, to officiate at the funeral. All were on their way to Santa Barbara within hours, or within a day.

My friend Grace couldn't decide which one of Stephanie's poems to choose for the In Memoriam leaflet she offered to design. She loved them all and then chose seventeen. This beautiful booklet in Steff's favorite color, pink, was Grace's last gift to my daughter—as it would be a gift to the mourners who received it during the funeral service.

She had so many friends, my Stephanie. Later they filled the little chapel at the Santa Barbara Cemetery and overflowed to the portico outside. Her life had touched those who knew her, and she was loved by them.

And I?

Her death wrapped me in opaque grayness. The California winter air, breezy and cool, seemed to withdraw from me—forcing me to take deep, deliberate breaths. My mind was blank. The blade churning in my chest was sharp. There are no words that can describe this pain. No words. My brain turned the phrase—*Stephanie, my dancing butterfly. Gone. Dead.*—over and over.

The word *death*, this terrifying word, should not have a connection to some-one young, to anyone's child.

I remembered when she wrestled with death, twenty-three years earlier, and she lived. I realized now, or perhaps rationalized, that these twenty-three years had been a gift to me—though often a struggle for her.

She had fought well, never giving up. She had reached a point in her life that satisfied her, having accepted certain limitations and having overcome others. Her life was about *ability*, not *disability*.

Within the last year she rarely asked, "Mom, if I had not been ill, do you think I could have gone to Harvard, like Dad? Would I be a writer, like you?"

I answered then, "You could have succeeded in many areas. You were born with many talents."

And now I tell you, Stephanie, your special gift, that which no illness could de-stroy, was your radiance, your love, your lightness of being."

It was late in the afternoon, and this was the last time I saw her. She lay sur-rounded by flickering candles and gold papier maché angels. She wore her fa-vorite red silk dress and her turquoise Navajo cross lay on her chest. It did not move up and down like a feather, as it had done when she had breath. My child, so still, so beautiful and seemingly asleep. I stroked the flow of her wavy hair, buried my face in it, inhaling its smell of citrus blossoms. As in life. Still show-ing sparks of gold in brown. As in life. I caressed her face, its skin, but it felt cold. I remembered the smooth river stones we used to collect in Red Rock. They had felt like that.

Her eyes were closed, dark lashes resting on her pale cheeks. I willed her to open them suddenly and their brown twinkle would beam at me mischievously —laughing, that she had fooled me once again. No, *this* was real. Stephanie was not playing games as in those times when I called her my Sarah Bernhardt. No, she would not open those eyes ever again. I bent to kiss her, no warmth came from her mouth. I swallowed hard. This time she was not coming back.

I turned and left. Softly I closed the door.

On our way home, Steven stopped the car. "Mother, look!" He pointed to a rainbow. It seemed to originate from Stephanie's cottage, spanning the sky with its arc, highest over my house—where we had lived such happy years—ending at the cemetery on the cliffs by the sea, where her ashes would be buried the next day. A double rainbow, bright, as I had never seen before. A rainbow of light so pure, with colors so intense, they numbed. I stared, until my eyes ached, and my face felt wet from rain and tears.

Her cremation is scheduled for seven. This evening her body will turn to ashes.

I cringed at the thought of Stephanie, my child, body of my body, going through fire.

Father Simon and we, who loved Stephanie, went to our beloved East Beach. We took Capri along. Many memories connected Stephanie to this place. Here, in an hour of dark despair, she had wanted to swim to the island far off in the mist, Anacapa. And here she had met Duane, with whom she found her last months of happiness.

The moon was full that night. It hung suspended from the cyan sky, lightly veiled by misting clouds, a metallic disk hovering high near the cliffs and swimming silver on dark waters. Father Simon looked at his watch: *it was time*. Our prayers for Stephanie rose to the sky, while her body at this hour was committed to the element of fire. Then Father Simon ended his prayer, saying, "Father in Heaven, please send us a sign that Stephanie has left her earthly form in harmony, that you and your angels have received her soul and she is at peace."

Capri turned, pointed, and let out a sharp bark. We turned with her and looked up to the sky. And there—a *moonbow* appeared. A diaphanous, wondrous sight, a translucent arc of light opposite the moon, spanning from the city—the house of cremation—to the sea. An arc made of soft lavender, turquoise, and silver.

And then I knew, Stephanie, that you were gliding over this moonbow-bridge and that your soul was free.

> I am a slave
> Inside my body
> God, lift my spirit high
> And let me be at peace with my soul
>
> I cry not
> For when I die I go as one
> Body, spirit, mind and soul
> Connected now
> Will then set free
> My spirit, mind and soul. . .
>
> —Stephanie Finell, October 6, 1994

The last six lines are engraved on Stephanie's headstone. Stephanie died January 11, 1995, at 7:30 p.m.

Chapter Thirty-One

Things a Mother Should Never Know

I read the coroner's report. A mother should not read the weight, in ounces, of her child's heart. Or learn the size of it. But I had to know what the report said about the medication in Stephanie's system. Had she forgotten to take her medicine? The report stated that no medication was found in her blood and sixty-eight Mebaral pills were left in her pillbox. This meant she had not taken any medication for at least three days, not since we returned from Ojai.

I remembered her casual nonchalance at the time, saying, "Love conquers all," and that Duane thought she might get along without her medicine. I repeatedly reminded her how important it was for her to take her pills. There was always the danger of a seizure. I thought she understood.

When I realized what had happened, I was filled with impotent rage. There was nothing I could do that could bring her back. Dr. Agnew told me that the position of her head and a slightly lacerated tongue, as mentioned in the coroner's report, indicated that Stephanie's death was caused by a violent seizure, which led to cardiac arrest. The coroner's autopsy report also confirmed Dr. Agnew's assessment of the PET scan, that her brain was filled with cysts.

Dr. Agnew and I had not discussed the result of the PET scan. The holidays had intervened, and when her death came, I did not know that something in her brain was found to be terribly wrong. The doctor later told me he was shocked when he reviewed the scan. He could not reconcile the devastation he saw on Stephanie's brain scan with the vivacious young woman he remembered from her office visits, where she appeared years younger, like an alert and lithe seventeen-year-old who joked and turned her fear of upcoming tests into humor. The PET scan revealed no hope, but Dr. Agnew still looked for confirmation as to his findings and sought opinions from several colleagues. He consulted with neurosurgeons, hoping that perhaps a possibility existed of surgically removing part of the affected brain. There had been cases where patients had lived quasi-normal lives with half of their brains removed. His colleagues' answers were negative. The cystic presence was too extensive. An operation would leave Stephanie without movement or language.

When I consulted with Dr. Agnew after Stephanie's funeral, I witnessed the impact her death had on him. His face, normally of a high color, looked ashen. His lips drew inward into a thin line, and his eyes were red. Had he shed a tear? Two long lines now engraved his otherwise smooth cheeks and were making his face sag. Never before had I seen a doctor look so sad and so moved.

On a later visit, on the model of a full-sized adult brain, Dr. Agnew showed me the parts where Stephanie's cysts had been located. The numbers on the measuring tape left nothing to conjecture. The cysts had replaced gray and white matter in the greater part of her left brain, as well as in a portion of her right. I learned that, with this large cystic presence in the cortex in both hemispheres (hollow, racquetball-sized holes described as *cystic degeneration* in the autopsy report), Stephanie would not have been able to live longer than six months. No medicine could have prevented her from having severe seizures or from becoming comatose again.

I could not reconcile any of this information. What exactly had caused the seizures. Were they caused by the cysts?

I learned that such destruction of brain tissue—in the autopsy report it stated that her brain weighed two-thirds and closer to half the weight of a normal brain—can lead to seizures, though neither the cysts nor the dead brain cells are in themselves the cause of seizures. The cells surrounding the cysts, which are in the process of dying, these damaged cells are irritable and can generate seizures. Once the damaged cells die, they no longer lead to seizures.

I am still puzzled as to how it was possible for Stephanie to write poetry until a day before her death, and how she had been able to exercise, sing, dance, and amuse the guests in the Oaks in Ojai spa a week earlier?

I thought of the brain as our most intriguing mystery organ again. I wondered how Stephanie had been able to regain so much function after her initial illness and coma? The explanation related to her age. When the Venezuelan equine encephalitis virus struck, the plasticity of her seven-year-old brain allowed surviving brain circuits to take over the role of those that no longer could fulfill their task. The right side of Stephanie's brain took over for the damaged left. She could function, but only on one side of her brain.

I was grateful I did not have knowledge of her condition and her prognosis during our years together, and especially that I did not know the result of the PET scan, which predicted her imminent death. She could not have been saved. Knowing her condition would have made our last weeks together unbearably painful.

Had she not died that January day, she might have drifted off into a twilight state never to fully awaken.

Days went by and then weeks. I felt as if I had opened the gates to an underworld of distorted shadows, where I encountered a landscape of desolation and despair, an endless gray, similar to my destroyed Berlin after the bombing and the end of World War II, when people walked the streets like zombies. At that time, I had been an observer. Now I was the zombie.

I waited for a phone call, just to hear her laugh, when logic told me there would be no such call. A week after her death out of habit I called her number, and the shock of her voice on the answering machine threw me down a black ravine into the hellfire of pain. I finally managed to climb out of these depths, but then my heart would do strange things: beat fast, skip a beat, flutter like a frightened bird, then slow to a quiet whisper of a thump. I wished my heart would simply stop. I longed to be with Stephanie. But, along with thoughts of death, came fear—the illogical fear that she was not coming back when I *knew* she was not coming back. The fear left me feeling nauseous, and I pushed my food aside.

At times irrational thoughts surfaced: *Let's run away to Greece together and drink ouzo in the Plaka. Remember Stephanie, how much you want to go to Greece?*

I spent hours sitting on a sandstone bench near her grave, staring out to sea, watching dolphins at play, herons coming home to roost in the Monterey Pines. I was hoping for solace from nature.

None came.

At night I longed to sleep, to dream of Stephanie, to see her once again if only as a shade, but even her shadow eluded me. Others dreamt of her, not I.

I envied mothers who had their child's father by their side when death struck. They could share their grief and lend each other comfort. Still, I had Aida and was grateful I could weep with her who loved Stephanie as though she were her American daughter. I had Martin. I had my friends, and I could bury my face in Capri's fur, Stephanie's dog.

A year passed. Occasional moments of light appeared. And I began to realize that Stephanie's death, as painful as it was for me, had come as a blessing for her.

I picked up her story, which I had begun writing some years earlier—the story of a mother and daughter battling through the ups and downs that illness brings, but never giving up and eventually finding happiness in Santa Barbara. Now the book would need a different ending. While writing about Stephanie, I began to feel her near me again. She whispered words into my ear, words of encouragement, words of love. I had found a way to connect with her, and it energized me. Through my words, Stephanie could be the teacher she always wanted to be and tell others how it feels to be brain damaged, and what it takes for a brain-injured person, one who is quite aware of her own condition, to face an often hostile world with grace and courage.

I once called her my butterfly girl, and laughing, she countered: "Yes, but a butterfly with a broken wing," referring to her paralyzed right arm. She then began to tell me a little story, saying she dreamt it, but her eyes twinkled and she smiled her impish smile:

The bumble bee watched the butterfly land near him on the petal of a rose. "How can you fly with a broken wing?" the bee asked. The butterfly thought for a while, moved her head toward her wing, and said, "I remember how I flew before and then I take off into the air and the wind carries me and I can fly up high into the sky."

The End

Postscriptum

Marvin Finell died in October 1998. He had suffered from progressive supranuclear palsy (PSP). It is a brain disease that takes years to develop, while in the interim it destroys part of the brain. In its early stages it mimics Parkinson's disease. It changes the person's personality and, with it, his behavior. Marvin suffered physically in the final stages, and there was no cure. I had forgiven him long before I learned about the dreadful disease he had contracted. I forgave him but wished I had known the causes of his behavior earlier. Mainly, I would have wanted Stephanie to know that her father, who hurt her so deeply on many occasions, had, maybe through his illness, become a changed man.

I have forgiven Judith, though at times I still have to battle negative thoughts.

Steven experienced his share of love—and love lost—until he found happiness with a sweet young woman, Melissa, with whom he has a second family. I now have a granddaughter, named Lily after my mother, Astrid-Lily, and another grandson, Aiden, born on my birthday in 2009, a year and a half after his sister.

Loren is in a loving relationship with a woman disabled by diabetes. He has lost both parents, and I worry about his future.

I lost touch with Duane, though others have seen him in town.

Father Simon died of a heart attack at age sixty-three, three years after Stephanie's death.

Having realized many of life's ups and downs, I have arrived at a place of tranquility and harmony. Martin is at my side, and I have time to write. I look out upon a beautiful garden he has planted, I watch yellow and orange butterflies wing among flowering bushes, and rabbits rustle beneath trees and the deer eat my roses. If Stephanie were here, she would love it all. But then, she is here, isn't she? kf